Rheumatologic Interviewing and

Physical Examination of the Joints

HOWARD F. POLLEY, M.D., M.S. in Medicine, F.A.C.P.

Senior Consultant, Division of Rheumatology, Mayo Clinic and
Mayo Foundation; Professor of Medicine, Mayo Medical School;
Formerly, Chairman of the Division of Rheumatology (1966–1976),
Mayo Clinic and Mayo Foundation, Rochester, Minnesota

GENE G. HUNDER, M.D., M.S. in Medicine, F.A.C.P.

Head of Section, Division of Rheumatology,
Mayo Clinic and Mayo Foundation;
Professor of Medicine, Mayo Medical School,
Rochester, Minnesota

SECOND EDITION

W. B. SAUNDERS COMPANY
Philadelphia   London   Toronto

W. B. Saunders Company: West Washington Square
                           Philadelphia, PA   19105

                           1 St. Anne's Road
                           Eastbourne, East Sussex BN21 3UN, England

                           1 Goldthorne Avenue
                           Toronto, Ontario M8Z 5T9, Canada

Library of Congress Cataloging in Publication Data

Polley, Howard Freeman, 1913–

Rheumatologic interviewing and physical examination of
the joints.

First ed. by W. P. Beetham and others published in 1965 under
title: Physical examination of the joints.

1. Joints — Diseases — Diagnosis.   2. Rheumatism —
Diagnosis.   3. Medical history taking.   4. Physical
diagnosis.   I. Hunder, Gene G., joint author.
II. Beetham, William P. Physical examination of the joints.
III. Title.   IV. Title: Physical examination of the joints.
[DNLM: 1. Joint diseases — Diagnosis.   2. Physical
examination.   3. Rheumatism — Diagnosis. WE544 P773r]

RC932.P64 1978   616.7'2'0754   77–16966

ISBN 0–7216–7279–5

Rheumatologic Interviewing and   ISBN 0-7216-7279-5
Physical Examination of the Joints

Last digit is the print number: 9   8   7   6

Preface
to the
Second Edition

This second edition of *Physical Examination of the Joints* has been renamed *Rheumatologic Interviewing and Physical Examination of the Joints* to reflect the extensive amplifications, changes, and additions. Like its predecessor, it is intended for physicians and students seeking an elementary yet comprehensive guide for the clinical examination and evaluation of patients with various rheumatic diseases. The details of this subject are still often overlooked or slighted in the medical school and graduate training of most physicians. Recognition of rheumatic diseases, however, is growing in clinical, investigational, and socioeconomic spheres. This is reflected by the increasing interest in these conditions exhibited by patients, their families, and therefore their physicians. Although therapy is not ideal for many rheumatic diseases at this time, careful and proper evaluation of the patient is a primary requisite for the development of better programs of treatment.

The favorable acceptance of the first edition has encouraged us to prepare this revised edition. Also, new or revised texts of rheumatology have given little attention to the essential details of the joint examination or the specific features characteristic of the rheumatic patient's history. New additions to our book include a chapter called "Interviewing to Obtain the History of Rheumatic Disease," a chapter on the cricoarytenoid joint, inclusion of data on the manubriosternal joint, additions of the techniques of muscle testing in seven chapters and revisions in three others; amplification of the chapters on the wrist, metacarpophalangeal and interphalangeal joints, spinal column, hip, knee, ankle and foot, and other less conspicuous but equally important corrections or additions throughout.

The detailed descriptions of joint examination techniques and other principles espoused in the preceding edition also have been continued. These include descriptions of pertinent anatomic features with intentional repetitions when they are a convenience to the reader and arrangement of the text according to objective signs rather than disease entities, which is in keeping with our primary concern for recognition and localization of disease and our secondary concern for diagnostic classification of disease processes. In addition, suggested readings are included at the end of the chapters for further information when desired, and most of them are new or updated.

The available pertinent literature again has been correlated with the experiences and concepts of the authors and other rheumatologists on the Mayo staff. We fully and gladly acknowledge and credit the important contributions to the first edition of Drs. W. P. Beetham, C. H. Slocumb, and W. F. Weaver. Their participation was vital to its completion and its success.

Mr. John M. Hutcheson, an important artistic contributor to the former edition, has provided 19 new anatomic illustrations and 32 new line drawings for this new edition, especially all of the additional line drawings to illustrate muscle testing. The Russell L. Drake drawings remain unchanged, and it may be of interest to note here that they constituted his last completed project prior to his retirement shortly before the first edition was published. We reiterate our thanks to the Section of Photography and to M. Katharine Smith for her editing of both the new and the former manuscripts so capably. In particular, we thank our colleagues in the Division of Rheumatology and in the Department of Orthopedic Surgery for assistance and support, especially Drs. J. J. Combs, Jr., Joseph Duffy, R. L. Linscheid, J. D. O'Duffy, and R. B. Tompkins for their critical reviews of certain of the new as well as former material. We also appreciate and record the capable assistance and patience of Mrs. Marilyn Riegler, who typed (and retyped several revisions) of our manuscripts.

Howard F. Polley

Gene G. Hunder

Preface
to the
First Edition

This monograph is intended for physicians and students who wish an elementary, comprehensive guide for conducting the physical examination of joints and for evaluating involvement of the joints in the various rheumatic diseases.

The technics of examination are described in detail, as the ability to perform the joint examination accurately is helpful and in most instances even essential for establishing the correct diagnosis. In discussion of the technic of examining joints only the pertinent anatomic features are presented. The anatomy of the synovial membrane is described in detail because it is of particular importance in the examination of the patient with an involved joint and because it is often poorly understood. Many non-articular physical signs present in rheumatic diseases are essentially part of general physical diagnosis; these are not described herein. Likewise the details of the history of the patient with rheumatic disease, important as they are in the evaluation and treatment of the patient, are beyond the scope of this undertaking.

The available medical literature has been correlated with the experiences and concepts of the authors and other consultants in rheumatology at the Mayo Clinic. At the end of each section describing the examination of a particular joint or a group of related joints, a list of references is supplied for those who may desire additional information.

The material in this text is arranged according to objective signs rather than disease entities. It is concerned primarily with recognition and localization of disease and only secondarily with the diagnostic classification of the disease processes. There is intentional repetition in the text for the purpose of relating anatomy to inspection as well as to palpation in the physical examination of the various joints and to minimize the need of cross reference as a convenience for the reader.

This monograph is the result of many persons' efforts. We are particularly indebted to Mr. Russell L. Drake and Mr. John M. Hutcheson, artists at the Mayo Clinic and the Mayo Foundation, for their contributions. Drawings of the joints, bursae, and synovial membranes were done by Mr. Drake and Mr. Hutcheson and the line drawings and range of motion charts were done by Mr. Hutcheson. We also wish to thank the Section of Photography for their help in obtaining many of the photographs. Miss M. Katharine Smith from the Section of Publications graciously and skillfully edited the manuscript.

William P. Beetham, Jr.
Howard F. Polley
Charles H. Slocumb
Walt F. Weaver

CONTENTS

chapter 1

Interviewing to Obtain the History of Rheumatic Disease

Despite continuing technologic advances in the diagnosis of rheumatic disorders, the patient's history remains the single most important diagnostic adjunct to the physical examination. Fortunately, there now is more awareness of the need to teach formal interviewing techniques, and the number of publications on the general subject of interviewing the patient is increasing. Methods described in these publications have been adapted liberally in this book as a guide for interviewing patients with rheumatic complaints. For more general discussions on interviewing, the references cited at the end of this chapter are recommended.

Details about the patient's musculoskeletal symptoms, obtainable only from the interview, are priceless in understanding the patient's illness. These details (1) define characteristics of the complaints as the patient perceives them, (2) suggest whether anatomically definable involvement is likely or not, and (3) permit evaluation of the patient's cooperation, motivation, and goals. Thus informed, the clinician may more readily achieve the objectives of accurate diagnosis and appropriate management, while dealing with the patient as a complete human being rather than merely as a case.

A diagnosis of arthritis or related disorders is often received by the patient with fear or apprehension, if not misunderstanding. Thus, the appropriate diagnoses should be considered carefully and established as accurately as possible before they are discussed with the patient.

HISTORY OF THE PRESENT ILLNESS

Chief Complaint

In the medical history, the present illness may be defined as the history of the development of the symptoms of the chief complaint. Indeed, the words *present illness* refer to all of the disease processes contributing to the patient's clinical condition at the time of the examination. The emotional aspects of patients' symptoms are often minimized (or overlooked) in medical school training. Since psychologic elements are especially important in chronic rheumatic diseases, the evaluation of emotional factors is emphasized in this presentation.

Obtaining the history of the present illness from a patient with rheumatic or musculoskeletal symptoms follows the pattern used in taking any other medical history but focuses on the involvement of the musculoskeletal system; that is, the symptoms associated with diseases, disorders, or disabilities of the organs of locomotion and the tissues of mesenchymal origin. The interview should be conducted in private and preferably in advance of the physical examination.

The object of the interview is to try to understand exactly what the patient means by what he says about his symptoms and their development. The history should encompass details of the symptoms, including their sequence and degrees, the acuteness, intermittency, chronicity, or rapidity of their courses, and patterns of progression, exacerbation, or remission; the effects of previous therapy, associated diseases, or stress;

and the ways in which the patient has been affected by the symptoms, including the specific character of existing disability.

Chronology is the most practical framework around which to organize the patient's rheumatic history, but the principle of flexibility should supersede any formal outline of procedure, whether traditional or problem-oriented records are utilized.

A valuable and informative introductory request is, "Tell me how you decided to come to see me at this time." When patients have not previously been asked this type of question, their answers may be delayed, sometimes until the end of the interview. In any event, if the question does not lead to a free-flowing, informative response, the physician may have to ask another question, as for example, "What symptom bothers you the most?"

The skilled interviewer encourages the patient to tell the story of the illness in his own way. This approach produces valuable information for the physician, even though it may be disjointed and incomplete, for he can note what the *patient* emphasizes and how the story is told and can recognize and evaluate nonverbal clues (see later section) as they occur. In general, the interviewer should restrain curiosity about any initially unmentioned details until an appropriate time that does not interfere with the patient's continuing spontaneity. Silence and listening are sometimes necessary techniques for persuading a patient to speak on his own.

When it becomes evident that the patient will not provide the needed information spontaneously, the interviewer begins asking questions more actively. Whatever his response, the patient should be encouraged to go into more detail without prejudice by the interviewer. Minor prompting of the patient often suffices. The interviewer usually should proceed from general subjects to specific subjects and should be as consistent as possible. Questions should be brief and simple, asked one at a time, and be designed to aid rather than impede the flow of information. (For example, "What did you notice next after the onset of . . . ?" or "Tell me more about. . . ."). Language should be as natural as possible for both patient and interviewer. Furthermore, listening and intelligent questioning by the interviewer may provide answers not to be found in the physical examination or by laboratory studies. An ever-changing chief complaint, for example, would suggest that significant emotional factors are involved. Repeated interviews are sometimes needed in dealing with complex diseases and with anxious, confused, or ill-prepared patients. In addition, findings from physical or laboratory examinations may indicate the need for more details.

Information about the anatomic regions and joints affected should be as precise as the patient's descriptions will permit. The site and distribution of the symptom, its onset, severity, and course, and the occurrence or absence of swelling should be included. A generally useful request is: "Show me exactly where you feel . . ." (use the patient's terminology for the discomfort described). Inquiry about the patient's ability to carry out the activities of daily living and about his social and vocational activities or limitations provides important information that often is not volunteered. Questions such as "How does it limit you?" or "What can't you do?" may help to define the degree of severity. In the case of injury, a precise account of the circumstances may be instrumental in determining the correct musculoskeletal diagnosis. Symptoms or disorders in other body systems also may contribute to the accuracy of diagnosis of musculoskeletal disease (see p. 9).

Experience and a knowledge of rheumatology will lead to the observation that some musculoskeletal symptoms and signs are common to more than one rheumatic disease. Symptoms relate as frequently to the structures that surround joints, such as tendons and muscles, as they do to the internal functions of the joints themselves. Symptoms caused by conditions *in* joints can indicate different diagnoses or therapies from those caused by conditions *around* joints. Physicians should accept the premise that patients may not be capable of telling directly where their trouble lies and may not see themselves as a product of their past life. They also are even less likely to appreciate that physiologic, pathologic, psychologic, social, and environmental factors are interacting concurrently to produce symptoms.

When a patient is unable to offer a satisfactory description of his complaint, it is acceptable for the interviewer to give him some adjectives to choose from without suggesting one to be of particular importance. What the patient talks about first may not be what bothers him the most. Failure to mention information may be an oversight but may also be due to denial or embarrassment. Such questions as "Is there anything else?" or "What else is on your mind?" may elicit further information.

The specific features of the patient's rheumatic symptoms should be pursued carefully and comprehensively and can be considered conveniently and appropriately in seven dimensions: (1) bodily location; (2) quality (like . . .); (3) quantity, including intensity, frequency, volume, number, size, extent, and impairment of function; (4) sequence, including time of onset, duration, periodicity, frequency, and course; (5) aggravating and alleviating factors; (6) setting in which the symptom developed; for example, whether the patient is alone, with others, or in a particular environment when the symptom is noticed; and (7) associated manifestations. These are essential data about symptoms, whether they are physical or psychologic in origin.

Another system for investigating rheumatic symptoms uses the "five W's": what, when, where, with whom, and why. *What* refers to the precise nature of the symptom — its quality, intensity, severity, and effect on activities of daily living. (The last-mentioned item may be related only partially to severity and disability.) *What* also includes any aggravating or alleviating factors. *When* relates to the time of both the first and later experiences of the symptom: how often and for how long it appears and when it recurs, improves, or worsens; *when* also refers to other things the patient may be doing when the symptom is experienced and just before and after it is noticed. *Where* inquires about the location of the symptom in the body, any change of location or radiation, and where the patient is when the symptom is experienced. The next question asks *with whom* the patient is when the symptom is felt and just before and afterward; it also asks how the symptom affects his relationships with these people. *Why* asks about the meaning of the symptom — organically, psychologically, and socially — to the patient, his family, and his job. It attempts to elicit circumstances associated with the symptom that might not be appreciated by the patient without specific inquiry. The interviewer should always encourage the patient to emphasize his reactions to and methods of dealing with the event, rather than simply asking about the event itself.

Previous Therapy

The *history of previous therapy* should be included either in the data on the present illness or in the past history. The individual, collective, and sequential effects of previous therapy on the course of the illness are important and are usually not volunteered by the patient. Medications being taken for presumably unrelated illnesses may also be important. This is well illustrated by the untoward effects on some patients of taking hydralazine or procainamide for cardiovascular diseases. If a treatment was tried and then abandoned, was it ineffective even though used properly? Did it cause side effects? Was the family uncooperative or was the patient uncompliant? Were other factors involved? What a patient says about previous treatment (and the physician who prescribed it) can help greatly in understanding and managing the patient. Previously successful treatment in chronic illness bodes well for the success of current therapy.

Patient's Behavior

Observation of a patient's behavior includes noticing his body movements, gestures, and vocal intonations. From these the interviewer may determine or at least form an opinion about whether a patient is reacting normally, aggressively, nervously, apathetically, or otherwise. The mask of words used at times by a patient to conceal a problem may thus be more readily recognized.

Body Movements. Body movements may reveal the patient's attitudes. Examples of those that may be observed during the interview and their possible interpretations include the following: The taking off of glasses by a patient may indicate that by thus blurring his vision he finds it easier to talk. Covering the mouth may suggest a patient's feelings of inadequacy. His words can be misleading, even erroneous, but his eyes and eyelids will show his true emotion. Rubbing hands together is considered a sign of anxiety. Movement of large joints with gestures flowing away from the body suggests excitement. Movement of small joints within the patient's body space suggests agitation. A depressed or fearful patient may shuffle without swinging the arms and turn the whole body instead of the head. Happy, trusting people move their arms freely outside of the body space and have a sharp, staccato rhythm when walking. When a fearful patient begins to relax, he may straighten up and lean toward the physician.

Speech. Emotion alters the normal voice through changes in pronunciation, emphasis, volume, timbre, pitch, and so forth. The higher the pitch, the more negative or uncertain the speaker probably feels. Anxious patients speak with tremulousness. Sad patients tend to speak at the end of exhalation. Angry patients may "attack" words. An observant, trained listener can recognize hostility, surprise, fear, or affection even when the speaker may be doing his best to disguise the emotion. Variations in speech may transmit information of which the patient is unaware.

Clues as to how a patient is feeling usually are conveyed by facial expressions that an examiner can learn to recognize. The most significant are expressions of anger, sadness, anxiety, and fear; a mask-like smile, embarrassment, shame, or disgust also may be important to recognize. Facial expressions can be important substitutes for an inability to express feelings verbally and may provide more accurate clues to true emotions than words do. Such expressions may be transient and subtle and partially concealed by culturally determined habits. Physicians also communicate nonverbally. If the physician looks concerned, puzzled, or even raises an eyebrow, the patient may think something has been said or done that is at least not "right." Physicians' remarks and behavior are never casual to anxious patients.

Attitude Toward the Illness. Determination of the patient's attitude toward the illness is needed to complete the history of the present illness. When direct questions are unproductive, nonverbal behavior or information offered indirectly — for example, whether the patient followed previously recommended therapy — can be informative. The interviewer can compare the disability he expects to find based on medical experience with the patient's own evaluation of the disability. Patients who complain of more or less impairment than seems appropriate may have a psychologic disorder that requires medical attention.

Arthritic or rheumatic illnesses and disabilities may lead to a legitimate state of dependency that is acceptable both to the patient and to those around him. Some patients who have returned to the infantile state of dependency find it exceedingly difficult to leave it. When there is little of satisfaction or substance to which to return, such patients may have little or no wish to do so. As noted by Morgan, the physician must try to understand the patient's fears both about the illness and about what may lie ahead after recovery, namely, the fears from which the illness may protect him. Sometimes recovery is delayed because the fear of being well overshadows the dissatisfaction of being ill.

Patients' attitudes toward their rheumatic condition may be closely related to their understanding of it. Patients often do not appreciate how their own behavior may modify a rheumatic illness or how behavior can be changed to aid recovery. Patients who come to a physician involuntarily at the insistence of relatives, friends, or other physicians are often less cooperative and thereby indicate an inability to accept responsibility for their recovery or for the maintenance of good health. The physician should be alert for reasons for the success or failure of any therapy and should look for signs of the patient's sense of personal responsibility (whether appropriate or inappropriate) for the illness.

PAST HEALTH

After the history of the present illness is elicited, the next portion of the interview is directed to the patient's past health. This part of the patient's history includes information about all previous major illnesses and injuries, especially those requiring medical attention or hospitalization. They are listed and described chronologically under five major subheadings: (1) general health; (2) childhood health; (3) adult health, including (a) medical illnesses, (b) surgical procedures, (c) psychiatric illnesses, and (d) obstetric history; (4) accidents and injuries; and (5) immunizations, allergies, and exposures to disease.

In the presence of chronic disease these categories may overlap, but the interviewer can arbitrarily resolve this. Information about past health usually can be recorded in less detail than information about the present illness, but it should be detailed enough that the physician can deduce, support, or refute the reliability of a previous diagnosis.

Sample questions might include, "Do you recall or have you ever been told that you have had anything like . . . before?" (Name the present symptoms.) Another could be, "Do you recall any injuries to . . . ?" (Name the part of the body.)

For patients with a rheumatic illness, the past history can reveal previous conditions pertinent to the present illness that were not appreciated as such by the patient or symptoms that were diagnosed differently before. Episodes of uveitis, bursitis, or renal colic are examples of conditions that may presage certain rheumatic diseases. Illness often arises from the stresses and strains of events that occurred earlier in a patient's lifetime, and these may be more influential in the present condition than the patient appreciates.

FAMILY HEALTH

A diagram of the family tree is a convenient way to record pertinent information regarding illnesses that might be related genetically,
psychologically, or environmentally to the patient's present illness. Negative information relating to the family history that pertains to the patient's present illness should also be noted.

Rheumatic disorders that occur in several members of the same
family may have a genetic basis, but environmental factors and the powerful effects of suggestion and imitation must not be overlooked, for
they may be significant. Children express the conscious and subconscious
impulses of their parents. Such attitudes may have been promoted so
subtly that an understanding of these interrelationships requires study of
both the child or adult patient and the parents. In treating patients who
are children, the interviewer tries to learn the attitude of the parents
toward the child's symptoms.

Rheumatic or other diseases that are likely to have occurred in
other members of a rheumatic patient's family include rheumatoid arthritis, gout, psoriasis, colitis, infections, predilections to degenerative joint
disease or spondylitis, rheumatic fever, and psychogenic musculoskeletal
conditions. The interviewer might ask: "Does arthritis or rheumatism run
in your family?" "Which family members had which diseases?", and "What
have you been told or what do you remember about . . . ?"

PERSONAL AND SOCIAL HISTORY

Inquiry into the personal history is often best delayed until the
more standard and less sensitive or threatening aspects of the rheumatic
history have been obtained. It is always advisable to give the patient time
to get used to talking about himself before discussing personal matters.
Valuable information initially withheld may be revealed after a relationship of trust has been established or after a patient has learned to appreciate the importance attached to the question by the physician. Often the
interviewer can reach areas of tension rapidly by recognizing and search-
ing for the gaps between the patient's desires and fulfillments. The in-
quiries about personal history should have relevance to the present illness, yet should be comprehensive enough to achieve optimal
understanding of both the patient and his illness.

Fruitful aspects of the personal history are (1) the patient's current
life situation and (2) his past development. The former is usually more
important and in some instances may have been included in the history
of the present illness. The developmental history becomes particularly
important in psychiatrically related illnesses.

Items to be considered in the present life situation are current living arrangements, family or other relationships that identify the significant persons in the patient's life, present occupation, economic status, and social and community affiliations and commitments. Also important are leisure activities (or their absence), special skills, patterns of sleep, dietary and other habits and use of time. Later inquiry should include more sensitive subjects such as the patient's basic personality, intelligence, satisfactions, pleasures, goals, ideals, philosophy, and manner of coping with stress. The interviewer must be cautious in categorically ascribing causality to past events. The emphasis should be on the patient's reactions and methods of dealing with the events and not simply on the event itself. The standard personal demographic data included in the personal history often will have been recorded routinely in advance of the interview.

Items to be considered about the patient's past development include childhood and adolescent events and educational, marital, and occupational histories.

Human beings differ more from each other in their values than in any other respect. What terrifies one person may be high adventure for another. Physicians must find out what is stressful to a patient and how it has become so. To varying extents, patients create their own environments, which in turn reveal the kind of person each one is. Responses to stimuli tend to become patterned and resistant to change. In any event, environmental forces, to which he must respond, act on a patient. These may be current or past forces or both. What a person wants to become influences to a great extent what he will become.

REVIEW OF SYSTEMS

The history is concluded with a review of systems. This is a final, systematic checking of other symptoms or minor illnesses that the patient may have had but has forgotten to mention. It includes past as well as current symptoms that were not considered part of the present illnesses and includes both positive and pertinent negative findings. The physician alone knows all the topics that should be discussed and has the larger responsibility for the comprehensiveness of the interview.

A significant saving of the interviewer's time may be realized by having the patient or a responsible relative record on printed forms in advance of the interview the patient's past development and family, personal, and social histories, as well as a review of systems.

Examples of revealing symptoms, diagnoses, or conditions that may be considered in a review of systems for patients with rheumatic symptoms are listed in Tables 1–1 through 1–6.

TABLE 1–1. REVEALING SYMPTOMS, DIAGNOSES, OR CONDITIONS OF THE SKIN AND MUCOUS MEMBRANES

Symptoms or Complaints	Diagnoses or Conditions
Rashes	Acrosclerosis
Canker sores	"Adiposis dolorosa"
Loss of scalp hair	Alopecia
Nail changes	Amyloidosis
Ulcers	Behçet's disease
Pallor; color changes	Calcinosis
Purpura	Causalgias
Pigmentations; sun sensitivity	Cutaneous infections; pyoderma
Nodules, tophi	Cyanosis; acrocyanosis; morphea
Contractures, tightening	Gout
	Hypertrophic osteoarthropathy
	Myositis ossificans
	Oculocutaneous syndromes
	Psoriasis
	Raynaud's disease
	Reactions to drugs or other chemicals
	Reticulohistiocytosis
	Scleroderma
	Sicca syndrome
	Stomatitis; vaginitis
	Thromboembolic phenomenon
	Vasculitis
	Xanthomatosis

TABLE 1–2. REVEALING SYMPTOMS, DIAGNOSES, OR CONDITIONS OF THE HEAD AND NECK

Symptoms or Complaints	Diagnoses or Conditions
Headache	Alopecia
Swollen neck glands	Behçet's disease
Loss of scalp hair	Cervical rib syndromes
Sore mouth, ulcers, canker sores	Gout
Neck pain or tenderness	Micrognathia
Difficulty in swallowing	Nasal ulceration or perforation
Painful eyes	Ochronosis
Photophobia	Oculocutaneous syndromes
Double vision, loss of vision	Optic neuritis
Tender scalp	Parotitis
Claudication of jaw	Psychoneurosis
Ocular or aural pigmentation	Relapsing polychondritis
Nodules, tophi	Retinopathy
	Scleritis, episcleritis
	Scleroderma
	Scleromalacia
	Sicca syndrome
	Temporal arteritis
	Thoracic outlet syndrome
	Thyroiditis
	Tracheal chondritis
	Uveitis, iridocyclitis
	Wegener's granulomatosis
	Xanthomatosis

TABLE 1–3. REVEALING SYMPTOMS, DIAGNOSES, OR
CONDITIONS OF THE CHEST

Symptoms or Complaints	Diagnoses or Conditions
Cough Painful chest Swollen glands	Aortitis Chondritis Endocarditis Interstitial pulmonary fibrosis Myocarditis Nodular pneumonitis Pericarditis Pleurisy Pneumoconiosis Pneumonitis Relapsing polychondritis Sarcoidosis

TABLE 1–4. REVEALING SYMPTOMS, DIAGNOSES, OR
CONDITIONS OF THE ABDOMEN

Symptoms or Complaints	Diagnoses or Conditions
Abdominal pain Peptic ulcer Painful rectum	Amyloidosis Hepatitis Inflammatory intestinal diseases Lymphoma Mesenteric vasculitis Pancreatitis Peptic ulcer Peritonitis Proctitis or proctalgia fugax Perisplenitis Splenomegaly Viral hepatitis

TABLE 1–5. REVEALING SYMPTOMS, DIAGNOSES, OR
CONDITIONS OF THE GENITOURINARY TRACT

Symptoms or Complaints	Diagnoses or Conditions
Painful urination Frequency or urgency of urination Bloody or cloudy urine Vaginal or penile discharge Flank pain Suprapubic or low abdominal pain Fever, chills Painful intercourse	Behçet's disease Cervicitis Cystitis Cysts Nephropathy Oophoritis Prostatitis Reiter's syndrome Salpingitis Sicca syndrome Stones Urethritis Vaginitis Venereal disease

TABLE 1-6. OTHER REVEALING SYMPTOMS, DIAGNOSES, OR CONDITIONS

Symptoms or Complaints	Diagnoses or Conditions
Fever with or without chills	Arteriosclerosis obliterans
Fatigue, malaise	Arteritis
Loss of weight	Bacterial endocarditis
Edema, swelling	Endocrinopathy
Claudication of extremities	Heritable disorders: connective
Numbness or other paresthesias	tissue and other disturbances of
Clubbing of nails	growth and development
Swollen glands	Hypertrophic osteoarthropathy
	Lymphoma
	Myositis ossificans
	Neuritis or neuropathy
	Neuroses, psychosis
	Raynaud's phenomenon
	Reflex neurovascular disorders
	Systemic infections
	Terminal (digital) angiitis

IMPORTANT SYMPTOMS IN RHEUMATIC DISEASES

Pain

Pain is the symptom that most commonly brings a rheumatic patient to a physician. The phenomenon of pain is complex and subjective and often extremely difficult to define, measure, and explain. Nevertheless, both the pain and the patient who has this symptom must be evaluated as accurately and objectively as possible. Most pain syndromes can be validated as well or better from the patient's history than from laboratory or x-ray examinations. Pain has different meanings to different people and even to the same person at different times. What the patient actually feels or experiences is more important than what the physician thinks he should be feeling. Responses to pain are affected by the person's current mood and emotional status, as well as by past learning and conditioning, basic personality, and the total present situation. A patient may imitate or learn (consciously or unconsciously) symptoms he sees in other people with pain problems.

Whether or not pain identifies a pathologic change in a specific organ or structure, it can serve to communicate a patient's helplessness in circumstances that may include unresolved or unappreciated conflicts. Some parts of the body are more sensitive to musculoskeletal pain than others. For example, although muscles do not have pain sensory organs as sensitive as those in the skin, muscles can be the source of severe, disabling pain when the metabolic products of physical activity (such as lactic acid) are not removed fast enough by the circulation. Physicians often fail to realize both how severely painful muscular spasms can be and that they can upset the person who has them emotionally as well as physically. The upset, in turn, may lead to further spasms and increased pain.

Analysis of a patient's rheumatic pain may be approached by using the outlines described on page 3. The details to be sought include the location, character, circumstances of occurrence and course, and associated factors.

Location. The anatomic regions, areas, or spots of pain, or the lack of anatomic correlation (as the case may be) should be described as precisely as possible. If the pain is in a joint, more likely than not an articular disorder is present. Pain between joints may suggest bone disease (with or without arthritis) or referred pain. Pain in bursal, fascial, or periosteal areas or along tendons, ligaments, or nerves may suggest disease in these structures. When pain is diffuse and without anatomic correlation to indicate an organ or structure, a functional rather than an organic rheumatologic problem may be suspected.

Because of overlapping innervation of articular and periarticular tissues, patients often describe their pain as occurring in the joints, but after careful questioning the pain will be found to be extra-articular in origin. Whether pain arising from a given structure is perceived by the patient as localized or diffuse may depend more on whether the tissue is superficially or deeply located than on the nature of the tissue itself. The distribution of deep pain corresponds with the segmental innervation of the deep structures rather than with the innervation patterns of the skin.

The patient often perceives pain that originates in the muscles of extremities as being in the joints when the segmental innervation of such joints and that of the muscles is the same. Pain in small joints of the hand or foot tends to be more accurately localized than pain in larger, more proximal joints such as the shoulder or hip, since the pain in these larger joints is more segmental in distribution.

Whenever patients give only vague or general descriptions of the location of pain, persistent and patient inquiry is necessary. For example, pain from the hip joint may be felt in the groin or buttock, over the greater trochanter, or in the anterior portion of the thigh or knee. If a patient complaining of "hip" pain does not volunteer specific locations, the interviewer must ask for more detail; and if the patient has pain in the areas mentioned above, specific inquiry about this pain must be made. Pain from the hip joint also can be referred entirely or partially to the knee (see p. 189).

Any changes in location of pain since its onset also should be elicited, because this information may be of diagnostic value. For example, the polyarthritis of rheumatoid arthritis may be continuous and progressive, in contrast with the typically migratory polyarthritis of rheumatic fever. The migratory polyarthritis of acute gonorrheal arthritis is often followed within days by a persistent monarthritic or pauci-articular involvement. The distribution pattern of polyarticular gouty arthritis can be clinically distinctive. Nonspecific synovitis followed by involvement of one or more distal interphalangeal joints in a patient with psoriasis can help to establish the presence of psoriatic arthritis. Involvement of one or both shoulders and hands but not of the elbows can indicate reflex dystrophy or the shoulder-hand syndrome.

Character. The interviewer should encourage the patient to describe the character of the pain in as much detail as possible; the word *pain* alone does not convey enough information. The quality or character may be sought by asking, "What does it feel like?" or "What kind of pain is it?" The interviewer also can encourage elaboration by comments or questions such as: "I don't understand." "Can you explain that some more?" "Anything else?" or just "And?" More specific questions may have the undesirable effect of interjecting the inquirer's own ideas or restricting the patient's description. If one must resort to suggesting descriptions of pain in order to obtain the information, it should be done without bias or leading questions that might convey what the interviewer thinks or wants to be told.

Pain may be described variously as from a negligible ache, a feeling of dullness, or tolerable hurting, straining, stiffness, or soreness to sharp, unbearable, excruciating, intractable, or intolerable. Pain may be steady, crampy, or throbbing; it may be felt as a pulling, boring, tearing or pressure; or it may be characterized by paresthetic manifestations that include burning, electric shock–like, prickling, numbing, pins-and-needles, or crawling sensations, to name a few. Pain of muscular origin may be described as a "pulled" muscle or ligament, a "charley horse," or "lumbago." Pain also can be described by analogy: "like a toothache (or migraine or labor pains)," "like a bruise (or sting or burn)," "like a stab with a knife," "like hitting my crazy bone," "like being in a vise," and so on. The words that the patient uses to describe the pain should be recorded, with a note stating whether the description was offered calmly or dramatically. The description is influenced not only by a given patient's impressionableness but also by his vocabulary and intelligence. Patients may say it is difficult or impossible to describe their pain. Although even this is a meaningful remark, they usually are able to describe the pain if their attention is focused appropriately on it.

Quality of pain usually is more significant than quantity. Assessment of severity or intensity often is difficult but usually can be achieved if patients appreciate the physician's sincere interest in and need for the details. Repeating the questions helps to emphasize the physician's interest. The duration, continuation, or intermittency of pain are other characteristics to be elicited.

As details of the description of pain are sought, the interviewer should pay particular attention to how the patient behaves and speaks. A description of agonizing or excruciating pain from a person not obviously in such discomfort should be properly noted and evaluated.

Circumstances of Occurrence and Course. The details of the circumstances associated with the patient's first awareness of the pain, whether the onset was gradual or sudden, what the patient thought was the cause, and how and what the patient feels as he is talking about it are to be sought. These can be elicited by questions such as: "Exactly what were you doing at the time you first felt the . . . ?", "Was it sudden or gradual in onset?", and "What makes it better or worse?" In particular, details to be looked for concerning aggravation include the effects of various body positions, movements, activity or inactivity, touch, pressure, and emotional stress. Important factors that may be contributing to relief or exacerbation also include drugs or other treatment being given.

The presence or absence of pain when at rest can be a critical point in the evaluation of patients with musculoskeletal disorders. Although there are exceptions, pain that occurs only during movement or motion may be described as mechanical. Pain both at rest and with movement is more suggestive of inflammatory, fatigue, or tension syndromes. The details of movement or activity can be elicited by questions about the patient's activities of daily living, use of analgesics (prescribed or otherwise obtained), and any physical therapy received (types, times). Special attention should be given to interactions or adverse effects of drugs. A patient may relate the onset of pain to an accident, although proper inquiry may determine that the patient had not been comfortable or functioned normally for some months or years before the accident or that a divorce or some other personal tragedy has a more significant temporal connection. Search for this information may begin with questions such as, "When did you last feel perfectly well?", "What was the significance of the [injury or stress] to you?", and "What did it do to your life, your marriage, your job, your self-image?"

The patient's anxieties (see following section), fears, and fantasies about the meaning of pain should be determined, along with whether the patient has known of other persons with a similar situation, why he thinks he has acquired such a symptom himself, and what memories or old emotional responses the symptom may evoke. Persistence or a change in the character of the pain from what it was at the onset should be clarified. Any change or other details of progression or regression should be elicited in chronological sequence, and whether the pain is actually present now, at the time of the examination, should be determined. Later an appropriate question may be, "Are there any benefits to you from this . . . [patient's adjectives]?" Pain can serve as a defense against failure and as a way to avoid the usually tolerable stresses of life. Chronic pain may protect a patient from more profound emotional or physical disintegration. Physicians must be aware that some patients with chronic illnesses, especially those characterized by chronic pain, may have no conscious desire or motivation to get well.

Associated Factors. The interviewer needs to determine how the patient reacts to the pain in terms of (1) local phenomena, such as related muscle spasm, paresthesia, weakness, Raynaud's phenomenon, or skin changes; (2) constitutional symptoms, such as autonomic dysfunctions, sweaty hands or feet, burning, numbness, and other types of paresthesia, loss or gain of weight, fever, chills, or interference with the activities of daily living at home, at work, and during recreational and other activities; and (3) emotional aspects. Students often are better trained to identify the anatomic and physiologic mechanisms that give rise to pain than to identify the psychologic, emotional, and social factors that help to answer the question, "Why did this illness strike this particular patient at this particular time?" Incongruity between what a patient says and what he does can alert the physician to suspect emotional instabilities. A neurotic or emotionally unstable person usually reacts more to relatively mild pain than a well-adjusted person does. Vague or dramatic answers suggest an hysterical personality; overly precise descriptions, an obsessive personality; and guarded, cautious answers, a personality with paranoid characteristics. An impulsive person may be demanding, impetuous, and plaintive. A patient with a passive dependent personality may have multiple symptoms and the desire to unload all decisions onto the physician. Characteristically, pain has no anatomic correlation when it is the result of a psychiatrically related hysterical or conversion reaction.

Depressed individuals usually are more susceptible to or less tolerant of pain than others. Depression can be a result of pain, a cause of it, or both. A depressed patient tends to be immobile and also is likely to be close to tears, with downcast eyes and unchanging, sad facial expression.

Anxiety and tension are overlooked too often as causes of pain. Pain, in turn, contributes significantly to or accentuates existing anxiety and tension. Anxiety may be acute, periodic, long-standing, or chronic.

Anxiety can be a result of injury to the body, changes of role, or separation — real, threatened, or fantasied. Patients complain of anxiety per se only infrequently. However, it is more commonly expressed in the form of concern about a particular organ or disease, which may be too disturbing for the patient to discuss directly. Other patients may complain of various symptoms of autonomic dysfunction, fatigue, insomnia, loss of appetite, or nervousness, or they may say, "I don't know why I feel the way I do." Previous episodes of anxiety may have resulted in other diagnoses, and responses to treatment in such instances may have been inappropriate. When anxiety is severe, patients probably have sought repeated examinations; the history of these can be informative.

Anger may be a patient's defense against anxiety, for anger allows him to manipulate the environment to obtain desired concessions and prevents development of the full discomfort of anxiety. The interviewer must not meet the patient's anger with his own. Rather he should try to learn what the patient is anxious about and what the anxiety means to the patient. This is often difficult, for it involves inquiring about the factors behind the anger or hostility and deciding whether the reaction is appropriate or not. A hostile person often has a grievance that is based on an unredeemed desire for acceptance. The grievance, however, is unlikely to be expressed for fear of further rejection. Such a person does not realize that his hostile manner significantly influences a self-fulfilling outcome.

Swelling

Swelling is an important symptom or complaint of patients with rheumatic diseases. Although assessment of swelling is certainly a function of the physical examination,* valuable information may also be obtained from the interview or from comparison of the patient's history with the physical examination. Swelling, whether present or absent, can be helpful in diagnosis, and asking about it is appropriate when a patient does not mention it himself.

Patients vary in their perception of swelling and in their ability to describe it. Thus, specific questions may have to be asked. Sample questions include: "Show me exactly where the swelling is," "When does the swelling occur?", "When the swelling is present, does the area look any different to you (or to others), or does it just feel different?" and "Does the swelling interfere with (or affect) any activities?" Swelling that is perceived only by the patient is called *subjective;* that which is visually or palpably demonstrable is called *objective.* An excess of fluid swelling in an anatomically distinctive compartment, such as the synovial sac or bursa, is described as an effusion.

Determination of the exact location of the swelling is essential, for it is necessary to know whether the swelling conforms to an anatomically discrete area. It is particularly important to know whether the swelling corresponds to a synovial, articular, or bursal distribution. Swelling may also be present in a diffuse or an anatomically distinct portion of an extremity or other part of the body or only in dependent parts. Inquiry regarding the symmetry of previous swellings is important. The patient may exaggerate the degree of swelling in a sincere effort to emphasize its presence, especially if previous interviewers have discounted or refuted the importance of a swelling that was perceived by the patient but that was not visibly conspicuous. Some patients, especially those who are obese, may interpret normal structures such as adipose tissue or even bony prominences as swellings.

Other information to be sought from the patient is whether the onset of swelling was acute or gradual and whether its course was intermittent or chronic. Questions should also be directed toward finding any ameliorating or aggravating factors the patient may have observed or suspected. These details usually are not obtained without specific inquiry.

The swollen area may or may not be painful. Discomfort may vary from an uncomfortable feeling, either at rest or during use of the part, to a dull ache with tenderness of varying degrees, to moderate, severe, or excruciating pain. Swelling in a confined area such as a synovial sac or bursa is usually worse during motion of a joint or of tissues that cause tension on the bursa. Swelling in such areas is most painful and tender when it has developed acutely. In such instances, even a light touch may be intolerable. In chronic

---

*See pages 34 to 36 and references to this aspect of physical examination in the various chapters on individual joints.

swellings when the synovial sac has stretched or when the distention has developed gradually, pain is mild or tolerable. Soft-tissue swelling outside contained sacs is less likely to be acutely painful. An exception to this may occur in emotionally labile, chronically tense, and fatigued hyperalgesic patients. Irrespective of the circumstances, the patient's perception of the degree of swelling as well as of the severity of the discomfort is worthy of notation.

Soft-tissue, and especially synovial, swellings should be differentiated from bony prominences that may have increased in size. Describing the latter as bony enlargements rather than as swellings eliminates the possibility of confusion or misinterpretation.

Soft-tissue swellings result from many conditions other than articular or rheumatic disorders (for example, from circulatory or metabolic disorders), which are beyond the scope of this discussion. Arthralgia or other musculoskeletal symptoms without swelling, especially when they are chronic, often strongly indicate the absence of articular disease.

Limitation of Motion

Limitation of motion is a frequent complaint of patients with rheumatic disorders. An insight into the extent of the disability resulting from lack of motion is provided by the patient's description. Patients often express such limitation in the context of the difficulties they experience from restrictions on their activities during work and daily living. Such information usually is readily elicited by questions such as, "What ordinary daily activities can't you do for yourself?" If further suggestion is needed, the interviewer may elaborate by asking if the patient can feed, clothe, or bathe himself, go to and from the bath and toilet without assistance, navigate stairs alone, and perform his usual work and other duties.

Patients also may describe limitation of motion as contracture, limping, or other abnormalities of gait or in terms of their awareness of other changes in physical appearance, but they rarely refer to themselves as deformed. The interviewer thus should avoid using the word *deformity* unless a patient has already used the term and is comfortable with it.

If there are restrictions of motion, the length of time they have been present should be determined as accurately as possible. The patient may have "kept going" despite the limitations and, if so, this also should be recorded. The date a patient may have quit employment, as well as the reasons for doing so, should be ascertained along with observations of any subsequent modification or limitation.

The type of motion restricted or lost may be active or passive (see p. 36). To a great extent this information is revealed by the physical examination, but interviewing can provide useful clues and may direct the attention of the interviewer by suggesting the type of motion lost even before the physical examination is made. Degrees of compensable limitation of motion and other functional classifications are available in orthopedic publications and are generally beyond the scope of this presentation.

Limitation of motion of a part of the body may be defined further as a loss of extension, flexion, rotation, or other motions, but this usually is determined more readily from the physical examination than from the history.

It is also helpful to determine whether the limitation of motion began abruptly (as in the case of a tendon or muscle rupture or a psychogenically related episode) or gradually and intermittently before becoming chronic. The effects of previous treatment also provide information that can be valuable for diagnosis and future therapy. It may be evident at the time of the interview whether any assistive devices, such as articular supports, canes, crutches, walkers, or wheelchairs, have been needed in the past or are currently required, but this is not invariably or always reliably true. A patient may come to the physician in a wheelchair for convenience rather than from need, and this may not be determined without specific questions. When a cane or crutch is used, the side on which it is carried should be noted. A patient carrying a cane on the side of the involved joint may do so from ignorance or because he does not need the greater assistive support provided when the cane is carried on the opposite side.

Limitation of motion may be complete in the presence of ankylosis or paralysis, but it is partial in most rheumatic diseases. Useful classifications of the degrees of restricted function in patients with rheumatoid arthritis have been published and are used widely in the study of patients with this disease.

Stiffness

The word *stiffness* has different meanings to different patients. Some equate it with pain, others with fatigue, soreness, aching, tightness, swelling, restrictive sluggishness, or weakness, and still others use the term without being able to describe clearly what they feel. Stiffness should be differentiated from the more persistent pain or other symptoms of arthritis. For this discussion, stiffness is defined as the discomfort, restriction, or both perceived by the patient when he attempts the first part of *easy* movement of a joint after a period of inactivity. Stiffness (when it occurs) usually develops after inactivity of one or more hours and often after a night's bed rest and sleep. When stiffness is mild, the patient may become limber in minutes. When severe, the stiffness may improve slowly over several hours or not improve appreciably. Stiffness may be noticed in localized, widespread, or scattered areas of the body, but usually it is not generalized, even though some patients may suggest that it is.

Stiffness formerly was considered a signal symptom of "fibrositis." Since this term has been applied to many seemingly unrelated rheumatic syndromes of both pathologic and psychologic origins with resulting confusion, the term is best discarded.

Stiffness is sometimes equated with *gelling*. That term has been used at times to refer more specifically to the stiffness which occurs after relatively short periods of daytime inactivity, in contrast with the more marked morning stiffness after a night's bed rest. Thus, although the word *gelling* is sometimes used, *stiffness* is the preferred terminology. Gelling is not listed or defined in medical dictionaries, and the nonmedical definitions do not encompass accurately the medical implications of stiffness.

Some patients who have rhematoid arthritis or other inflammatory articular disorders, such as polymyalgia rheumatica and ankylosing spondylitis, are sufficiently capable observers that they can describe their stiffness concisely, readily, and accurately. With other patients, more tedious inquiry is required to determine its presence or absence. Evaluation of a patient's complaint of stiffness often can be one of the most difficult tasks encountered in interviewing for rheumatic diseases. In all instances, it is important first to find out whether stiffness is present or absent and second, if it is present, to understand what stiffness means to the patient without asking leading questions. If a patient has not been asked previously to define the stiffness in his own words and in detail, a satisfactory or interpretable answer may not be obtainable. In such instances, the patient should be re-questioned after he has taken the time (perhaps a week or two) to make the pertinent observations concerning the consistency or variability of his stiffness.

Bona fide morning stiffness can be a prodromal sign of arthritis. It is the first of the diagnostic criteria for rheumatoid arthritis listed by the American Rheumatism Association, and it is usually considered a hallmark of the inflammatory processes of the disease. To merit this consideration, the stiffness of inflammatory articular diseases should be differentiated from that of mechanical, degenerative, or destructive joint diseases. The stiffness of these generally noninflammatory joint diseases is almost always of shorter duration (usually less than one-half hour) and of lesser severity than the stiffness of inflammatory joint disease. In mechanical, degenerative, or destructive joint diseases, the stiffness is temporally related to the extent of overuse of the damaged joints and responds, usually within a few days, to adequate limitation of the use of joints.

The absence of stiffness does not exclude the possibility of the presence of systemic inflammatory rheumatic diseases such as rheumatoid arthritis, but such absence is uncommon. Stiffness from neurologic disorders of the Parkinson type, without a recognized inflammatory basis, also occurs and sometimes is conspicuous, although the "limbering" component is lacking. Other characteristic differential clinical features help to clarify the diagnosis.

Attempts have been made to simplify the interview on the subject of stiffness by asking a single question such as "Are you stiff on arising?" or "Do you wake up with stiffness or aching in your joints or muscles?" Use of either question may helpful for general screening purposes; however, oversimplifying circumvents the purpose of the interview and the answers can be misleading.

It is important that the interviewer take the time and have the patience to ask the precise questions that may be necessary to determine whether a patient has morning stiffness, because the information obtained may influence a decision with regard to the diagnosis or the exclusion of articular disease. The presence and duration of morning stiffness are related to (1) the duration and (2) the quality of sleep.

Certain questions will help develop the required information. The first question is, "At what hour do you usually go to bed?" "This is followed by, "Do you go to sleep right away?" and if not, "What time do you go to sleep?" Next, "Do you sleep well?" or "Are you awakened in the night?" If so, "At what hour?" and "What do you do when this happens?" "Do you take aspirin or other medicine?" "Do you get out of bed?" "How long are you up?" "How long before you go back to sleep?" "How long do you sleep again after being awakened?" "What time do you wake in the morning?" Many times it is helpful to relate these questions to a definite date or time, such as the previous night, so that the patient can remember well enough to give the necessarily detailed replies.

After establishing these preliminary details, the critical question is, "How do you feel when you first awaken, while you are still lying quietly in bed and before any movement of the joints?" If the patient has been awake in the night, a comparison of the feeling at that time with that in the morning is also valuable in assessing stiffness. Other related questions in either instance include, "Are you comfortable or not?" and "Do you feel rested or tired?"

The patient with rheumatoid arthritis usually is comfortable and rested after sleeping well on first awakening and before any movement. The next question, therefore, is, "What, if anything, do you have to do in the morning to know whether or not you are stiff?" This question may have to be elaborated upon if the patient does not understand how to answer. Then it is necessary to amplify it by asking, "Do you need to move to become aware of the stiffness and, if so, how much do you have to move?"

The interviewer then proceeds to find out about the first *easy* (gentle) movements. It is helpful to select a single joint, such as the knee, or a part of an extremity, such as a hand or foot, and ask specifically how the designated joint or joints feel with the first easy motions, such as drawing the knee up *part way* or straightening it out if it was partially flexed on awakening or using a hand to move the bed covers, as contrasted with attempts at making a tight fist. This question is followed by, "How does this feeling compare with that observed at rest, before any motion?"

The inflammatory tissue reactions to which morning stiffness is attributed cause the patient with rheumatoid arthritis or related disorders to note more discomfort with the first easy motions than at rest. In contrast, stiffness related to fatigue or tension is present on awakening before any motion and the first *easy* motions may change the amount or character of discomfort only slightly, if at all. Their increased discomfort occurs at the extreme of the range of motion.

The interviewer then asks the patient whether he has symptoms as he moves into the upright sitting position on the side of the bed, before any weight bearing. Generally, stiffness with this activity is the same as that ascribed to the first easy motions made while the patient is still resting in bed. It may, however, be increased.

Then the question is asked, "How do the joints feel during the first few steps away from the bed?" The physician determines how this reply, concerning the stiffness or discomfort felt during this fraction of the early morning activities, compares with the one previously elicited about discomfort during motion while at rest in bed and during the later, more active processes of dressing, descending stairs, and other morning activities. Morning stiffness that is accentuated primarily or only by these later, more active weight-bearing activities is not characteristic of the inflammatory type of stiffness seen in rheumatoid arthritis.

The final question then is, "How long does it take you to become as limber as you are likely to be for the day?" This period of time usually varies from day to day, and a record of the usual range is a more reproducible type of data than is a single or average time period.

The next aspect of stiffness to be elicited is its location. A simple question such as "Where does the stiffness occur?" usually suffices. This information is often volunteered by the patient or can be elicited initially in order to help focus on the description and the definition of what the patient means by stiffness. Usual sites are the joints and periarticular tissues which are affected by the arthritic process. Common areas are the neck and shoulder girdle, hands, and low back; areas peripheral to, around, or between other joints; and the muscular and fleshy parts of extremities between joints. In patients with widespread articular or related disorders, bilateralism is more usual than unilateralism. The latter, however, can be encountered when the inflammatory process is more localized, as for example, in a monarthritis or a periarticular area such as the shoulder.

Other details of occurrence include the diurnal pattern, if any, the degree of severity, persistence, or recurrence, the effects (if any) on activities of daily living, and the effects of daytime inactivity. The last mentioned item should also be assessed by details of time, position, condition upon awakening, and relation to activity, as morning stiffness is. "Does it clear up, improve, or remain static?" Stiffness caused by inflammatory conditions usually is not present all day; stiffness related to fatigue and neuromuscular tension may be.

Changes in environmental temperature, humidity, barometric pressure, or other discernible features of weather can influence stiffness or its symptomatic onset or duration. These vary from patient to patient. The effects of the previous day's activities, of air conditioning and heat therapy (including hot tub baths), and of physical or emotional strain are pertinent to an accurate, detailed evaluation of symptoms. Patients who are irritated or frustrated by persistent attempts to obtain the details of stiffness or who are consistently vague about them are less likely to have the morning stiffness associated with inflammatory rheumatic disorders. Inquiry about fatigue (see p. 24) is best made separately. Otherwise, the patient might confuse the two symptoms.

The details about morning stiffness may be easier to obtain if the patient temporarily omits taking salicylate or other anti-inflammatory drugs or is given a sedative at bedtime. Either or both should increase the morning stiffness of a patient who has rheumatoid arthritis, whereas a sedative given to a patient with nervous fatigue usually will induce a better night's rest and result in much less or none of the usual so-called (but false) morning stiffness. The morning stiffness of some patients may also be ameliorated by a significant elevation of the body temperature.

Stiffness has some relationship and similarity to limitation of motion but differs from it by being either a more subjective symptom or an objective but transient difficulty in achieving range of motion rather than a persisting problem. Limitation of motion more precisely describes a continuing, albeit not necessarily permanent, deficit (see p. 36).

Weakness

Weakness is a loss of motor power or muscular strength. When present, it is nearly always objectively demonstrable during examination, at least in relation to what a patient formerly was able to do. Muscular weakness causes a decreased capacity to perform work. True weakness can be noticed only when muscles are actually being used. In musculoskeletal disorders, weakness usually is persistent rather than intermittent unless accompanied by fatigue, and it frequently is associated with other evidence of severe physical illness, such as weight loss and fever. When weakness is marked, the patient may need assistive devices such as canes, crutches, a wheelchair, or other types of assistance to perform the activities of daily living. Grip strength, shoulder and neck function, ability to chew and swallow, and ocular, respiratory, bladder, and bowel control all may be diminished by weakness, although these changes are sometimes less conspicuous than difficulties in ambulation or weight-bearing. Patients with myopathies marked by weakness have little or no difficulty in identifying the muscular system as the site of the weakness and usually can differentiate readily their muscular weakness from the more general symptom of fatigue. Muscular weakness as a result of inflammatory myopathies occurs most typically in the proximal parts of the extremities, whereas the weakness caused by most neuropathies is found in the distal or peripheral parts.

Weakness can also be a subjective symptom. It can be confused by the interviewer with other symptoms if the patient's description of its location is imprecise or misunderstood. Incisive questioning can elicit more exact information. Occasionally, patients may confuse weakness with stiffness. In cases of stiffness, pain, not lack of strength, limits motion. Weakness probably is most often confused with fatigue, although fatigue or other combinations of symptoms may indeed coexist. Difficulty in distinguishing symptoms can also be encountered when patients are vague observers or narrators, are self-flattering, or are inclined to rationalize and say they are weak when they really mean they are tired.

Weakness may be a sign of articular disease, myositis, and other types of myopathy, or of neurologic conditions.

Fatigue

Fatigue, although a common and important complaint of many patients with musculoskeletal disease, is an imprecise term. There is as yet no standard definition of fatigue, but it can describe either a generalized normal response to stress over a period of time or a decreased level of vitality resulting from complex biologic phenomena. The factor of time is particularly important in both the development and the resolution of fatigue. Normal or acute fatigue is a well-known, if not universal, human experience that disappears after a relatively short but adequate period of rest. When normal rest, recreation, and sleep are insufficient to restore a patient's depleted energies, chronic or cumulative fatigue results and may become clinically significant by limiting or modifying the patient's ordinary daily activities. Although the cumulative effects of events predisposing to fatigue are important when present, the factors that result in chronic fatigue permeate the total life pattern of the person affected.

The neurophysiologic manifestations of fatigue simulate the effects of sleep deprivation. These include decreases in attention, perception, and motivation, and in the ability to perform other mental and physical activities; a depressed mood or affect; general restlessness or irritability; and an increased sense of tiredness with a desire for sleep but the inability to obtain it. In the absence of organic disease, anxiety and muscular tension or related emotional states are prominent factors in producing chronic fatigue, but significant individual differences preclude prediction of the precise circumstances that will induce chronic fatigue.

When fatigue is stressed particularly by a patient, it may be an early or prominent symptom of significant illness or have important psychologic meaning for the person.

Fatigue is a complaint of patients with either inflammatory or functional rheumatic syndromes. Patients may describe this symptom in terms of feeling tired, weary, "all in," or worn-out; as a lack of pep or interests; or as listlessness, stiffness, or weakness. The patient appears lethargic, with slumped posture, sagging or sad facial expression, and a dull, toneless voice. When fatigue is perceived primarily in muscular tissue, it may be confused with weakness. The differentiation between stiffness and weakness is especially important. It may be facilitated by considering fatigue as a disinclination to activity or movement, stiffness as a discomfort during movement or activity, and weakness as an inability to move.

Fatigue may be felt when the patient is resting after muscular or neuromuscular activity but has not yet rested enough to have recovered. In contrast, weakness is noticed only when muscles are actually being used. Patients with articular disease associated with muscular weakness and atrophy may fatigue easily or be continuously fatigued.

Evaluating a complaint of fatigue requires consideration of the factors of time, activity or inactivity, the presence or absence of anxieties, and the patient's sense of well-being. Both physical and psychologic factors should always be considered. The interviewer needs to learn how many hours the patient spends in bed during an ordinary 24-hour period, the time of day fatigue is perceived, the quality of and response to rest and sleep, whether fatigue is present upon sitting and reclining or only upon ambulation or both, the length of time fatigue has been present, the nature of its course during this interval, and whether its onset was sudden or gradual. Sometimes fatigue is unaccompanied by objective evidence of disease, is experienced suddenly, or is characterized by considerable and even impetuous variability, both in degree and in its response to distracting or enticing stimuli. In such cases, precipitating emotional factors are likely to be involved, and must be determined, especially if the patient fails or is reluctant to appreciate the correlation.

Fatigue is commonly associated with other symptoms of articular or neuromuscular disease and may be a prodromal symptom of inflammatory types of arthritis. This relationship, however, can in many cases be elicited only by direct or more often by retrospective inquiry. Fatigue has been considered by some to be a reliable index of the inflammatory processes of rheumatoid arthritis, one that can be assessed with less observer error than the duration of morning stiffness, probably because patients usually can be more precise in their recognition of its time of onset and duration. Occasionally, however, fatigue may be only vaguely and nonspecifically definable or even absent in rheumatoid arthritis or in other conditions with which it may be associated.

SUGGESTED READING FOR ADDITIONAL INFORMATION

1. Engel GL, Morgan WL Jr: Interviewing the Patient. Philadelphia, WB Saunders Company, 1973, 129 pp.
2. Froelich RE, Bishop FM: Clinical Interviewing Skills: A Programmed Manual for Data Gathering, Evaluation, and Patient Management. Third edition. St. Louis, CV Mosby Company, 1977, 176 pp.
3. MacBryde CM, Blacklow RS (editors): Signs and Symptoms: Applied Pathologic Physiology and Clinical Interpretation. Fifth edition. Philadelphia, JB Lippincott Company, 1970, 1025 pp. (especially Chapters 1, 3, and 12).
4. Bonica JJ, Procacci P, Pagni CA (editors): Recent Advances on Pain: Pathophysiology and Clinical Aspects. Springfield, Ill. Charles C Thomas, 1974, 373 pp.

chapter **2**

Introduction to Physical Examination of the Joints

The ability to recognize what can be seen is a rewarding diagnostic dividend. Since the joints and other musculoskeletal structures are derived from the mesenchyme, which is characterized by a potential for marked cellular reactivity in the presence of disease, and since many of these are near the surface of the body, the observing examiner is provided an excellent opportunity for obtaining significant information about many diseases.

To help detect and localize disease within or outside of the joint, the techniques of physical examination of the joints and related structures will be correlated with articular anatomy throughout this monograph. The details of such examination are particularly helpful in analyzing the symptoms and signs of the rheumatic component of diseases which are localized to an articular area or to the musculoskeletal system or may be an expression of generalized or systemic diseases.

Accurate diagnosis as well as adequate care of the patient with articular disease also requires a complete general medical examination in addition to thorough study of the joints and adjacent tissues. The value of careful physical examination of the joints and related musculoskeletal structures is indicated by the broad spectrum of diseases and conditions that symptomatically and objectively affect joints; this is illustrated by the variety of diseases included in the following nomenclature and classification of arthritis and rheumatism, which was recently updated in the seventh edition of the *Primer on Rheumatic Diseases,* published under the auspices of the American Rheumatism Association Section of the Arthritis Foundation. Knowledge of the conditions in this list can aid the examining physician in considering the diagnostic possibilities in individual patients.

AMERICAN RHEUMATISM ASSOCIATION NOMENCLATURE AND CLASSIFICATION OF RHEUMATIC DISEASES*

I. Polyarthritis of unknown etiology
   A. Rheumatoid arthritis
   B. Juvenile rheumatoid arthritis (including Still's disease)
   C. Ankylosing spondylitis
   D. Psoriatic arthritis
   E. Reiter's syndrome
   F. Others
II. "Connective tissue" disorders (acquired)
   A. Systemic lupus erythematosus
   B. Progressive systemic sclerosis (scleroderma)
   C. Polymyositis and dermatomyositis
   D. Necrotizing arteritis and other forms of vasculitis
      1. Polyarteritis nodosa
      2. Hypersensitivity angiitis
      3. Wegener's granulomatosis
      4. Takayasu's (pulseless) disease

*Reprinted with permission from the Primer on Rheumatic Diseases. Prepared by a committee of the American Rheumatism Association Section of the Arthritis Foundation. JAMA, *224* (Suppl 51):16–17, 1973.

     5. Cogan's syndrome
     6. Giant cell arteritis (including polymyalgia rheumatica)
   E. Amyloidosis
   F. Others
     (See also Rheumatoid arthritis, I. A; Sjögren's syndrome, VI. G)
III. Rheumatic fever
IV. Degenerative joint disease (osteoarthritis, osteoarthrosis)
   A. Primary
   B. Secondary
V. Nonarticular rheumatism
   A. Fibrositis
   B. Intervertebral disk and low back syndromes
   C. Myositis and myalgia
   D. Tendinitis and peritendinitis (bursitis)
   E. Tenosynovitis
   F. Fasciitis
   G. Carpal tunnel syndrome
   H. Others
     (See also Shoulder-hand syndrome, VIII. C)
VI. Diseases with which arthritis is frequently associated
   A. Sarcoidosis
   B. Relapsing polychondritis
   C. Schönlein-Henoch purpura
   D. Ulcerative colitis
   E. Regional enteritis
   F. Whipple's disease
   G. Sjögren's syndrome (sicca syndrome)
   H. Familial Mediterranean fever
   I. Others
     (See also Psoriatic arthritis, I. D)
VII. Associated with known infectious agents
   A. Bacterial
     1. Gonococcus
     2. Meningococcus
     3. Pneumococcus
     4. *Streptococcus*
     5. *Staphylococcus*
     6. *Salmonella*
     7. *Brucella*
     8. *Streptobacillus moniliformis* (Haverhill fever)
     9. *Mycobacterium tuberculosis*
   10. *Treponema pallidum* (syphilis)
   11. *Treponema pertenue* (yaws)
   12. Others
     (See also Rheumatic fever, III)
   B. Rickettsial
   C. Viral
     1. Rubella
     2. Mumps
     3. Viral hepatitis
     4. Others
   D. Fungal
   E. Parasitic
VIII. Traumatic and/or neurogenic disorders
   A. Traumatic arthritis (the result of direct trauma)
   B. Neuropathic arthropathy (Charcot joints)
     1. Syphilis (tabes dorsalis)
     2. Diabetes mellitus (diabetic neuropathy)
     3. Syringomyelia
     4. Myelomeningocele

      5. Congenital insensitivity to pain (including familial dysautonomia)
      6. Others
   C. Shoulder-hand syndrome
   D. Mechanical derangement of joints
   E. Others
      (See also Degenerative joint disease, IV; Carpal tunnel syndrome, V. G)
IX. Associated with known or strongly suspected biochemical or endocrine abnormalities
   A. Gout
   B. Chondrocalcinosis articularis ("pseudogout")
   C. Alkaptonuria (ochronosis)
   D. Hemophilia
   E. Sickle cell disease and other hemoglobinopathies
   F. Agammaglobulinemia (hypogammaglobulinemia)
   G. Gaucher's disease
   H. Hyperparathyroidism
   I. Acromegaly
   J. Thyroid acropachy
   K. Hypothyroidism
   L. Scurvy (hypovitaminosis C)
   M. Hyperlipoproteinemia type II (xanthoma tuberosum and tendinosum)
   N. Fabry's disease (angiokeratoma corporis diffusum or glycolipid lipidosis)
   O. Hemochromatosis
   P. Others
      (See also Inherited and congenital disorders, XII)
X. Neoplasms
   A. Synovioma
   B. Primary juxta-articular bone tumors
   C. Metastatic malignant tumors
   D. Leukemia
   E. Multiple myeloma
   F. Benign tumors of articular tissue
   G. Others
      (See also Hypertrophic osteoarthropathy, XIII, I)
XI. Allergy and drug reactions
   A. Arthritis due to specific allergens (e.g., serum sickness)
   B. Arthritis due to drugs
   C. Others
      (See also Systemic lupus erythematosus, II, A, for Drug-induced lupus-like syndromes, e.g., hydralazine and procainamide syndromes; Hypersensitivity angiitis, II, D. 2)
XII. Inherited and congenital disorders
   A. Marfan's syndrome
   B. Homocystinuria
   C. Ehlers-Danlos syndrome
   D. Osteogenesis imperfecta
   E. Pseudoxanthoma elasticum
   F. Cutis laxa
   G. Mucopolysaccharidoses (including Hurler's syndrome)
   H. Arthrogryposis multiplex congenita
   I. Hypermobility syndromes
   J. Myositis (or fibrodysplasia) ossificans progressiva
   K. Tumoral calcinosis
   L. Werner's syndrome
   M. Congenital dysplasia of the hip
   N. Others
      (See also Arthropathy associated with known biochemical or endocrine abnormalities, IX)
XIII. Miscellaneous disorders
   A. Pigmented villonodular synovitis and tenosynovitis
   B. Behçet's syndrome

C. Erythema nodosum
D. Relapsing panniculitis (Weber-Christian disease)
E. Avascular necrosis of bone
F. Juvenile osteochondritis
G. Osteochondritis dissecans
H. Erythema multiforme (Stevens-Johnson syndrome)
I. Hypertrophic osteoarthropathy
J. Multicentric reticulohistiocytosis
K. Disseminated lipogranulomatosis (Farber's disease)
L. Familial lipochrome pigmentary arthritis
M. Tietze's syndrome
N. Thrombotic thrombocytopenic purpura
O. Others

EXAMINATION OF THE JOINTS

The physical examination of the arthritic patient actually begins when the physican first sees the patient and obtains useful information from the general appearance and attitudes of the patient, gross deformities, state of nutrition, gait, and body position. For example, observations can be made of the patient's ability to get out of a chair or bed, to climb up or down stairs, to care for himself, and to perform the usual daily functions such as feeding, writing, and dressing. Information regarding function of muscles and joints is obtained from, and should be included in, the inquiry into the patient's history.

In the clinical evaluation of joints the variations among individuals without definite articular abnormalities are of interest and should be considered. The only really reliable method of learning how to examine joints and of remaining familiar with the variations of normality is by repeated experience. The examiner must be aware of the variations produced by age, sex, body habitus, and occupation as well as those resulting from heredity and disease.

Structure and Classification of Joints

Interpretation of the examination of joints is facilitated by an understanding of the significant anatomic aspects of the joints of the body. Joints or articulations are formed wherever bones of the skeleton are joined to one another.

Joints are of three main types: (1) synarthroses (immovable articulations), (2) amphiarthroses (slightly movable articulations), and (3) diarthroses (freely movable articulations). In synarthrotic joints the bones are joined and held together by continuous intervening layers of fibrous tissue or cartilage. The surfaces of the joined bones are in almost direct contact with each other, and this close contact allows no appreciable motion. The joints between the bones of the skull are examples of synarthroses. The bony surfaces of amphiarthrotic joints are united by fibrocartilaginous disks, as in the articulations between vertebral bodies, or are joined by a fibrous interosseous ligament, as in the inferior tibiofibular articulation. Diarthroses are freely movable joints lined with synovial membrane in which the bones are separated from each other by a fluid-containing cavity. The knee joint is an example. Diarthrodial joints are the most common joints in the body and are the joints with which the rheumatologist is particularly concerned. In this and subsequent chapters the term *joint* will refer to a diarthrodial joint, unless otherwise stated.

The articulating ends of the bones forming a diarthrodial joint are covered by cartilage and are enclosed in a capsule of fibrous tissue. The joint capsule is strengthened by strong ligaments extending between the bones of the joint. The articular cartilage, which normally is resilient, acts as a cushion between the bones, and the smooth surface of the cartilage allows ease of movement. The synovial membrane lines the inner surface of the fibrous capsule, forms the inner lining of the joint, and is attached at the margins of the articular cartilages. The synovial membrane between these margins is composed of folds and pouches which facilitate or allow movement of the joint (Fig. 2–1). Normally only a

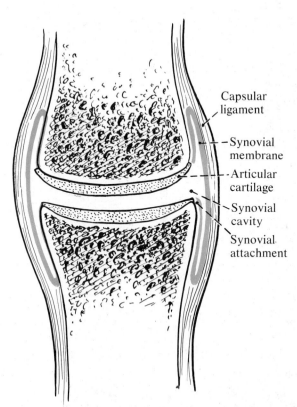

Capsular
ligament

Synovial
membrane

Articular
cartilage

Synovial
cavity

Synovial
attachment

Figure 2–1. Schematic diagram of a typical diarthrodial joint. Synovial membrane is shown in blue.

small amount of synovial fluid is present within the confines of the synovial membrane to provide lubrication for the inner surface of the joint. The volume of synovial fluid varies somewhat from joint to joint, but even in the largest peripheral joint (the knee) the recoverable volume normally can vary from none, in cases in which no free fluid can be aspirated although the surfaces of the joint are moist from a thin layer of viscous fluid, to about 3.5 ml of free fluid. Diarthrodial joints have an exceedingly low coefficient of friction.

Diarthrodial or synovial joints have been classified further according to the shapes of the surfaces that articulate. The shape of the articulating surface, in turn, determines the type and extent of motion in the joint. According to Barnett and associates there are seven types or forms of articulating surfaces: plane, spheroidal, cotylic, hinge, condylar, trochoid, and sellar. This descriptive classification was adopted and recommended for general use by the Sixth International Congress of Anatomists in Paris in 1955.

Plane Joints.   Plane joints allow only gliding movements. Gliding movement is the simplest type of joint movement that can take place and consists of one surface moving over another without any rotatory or angular movement. Articular surfaces of this type of joint are supposed to be planar or flat. Actually they are often slightly curved. The slight movement in this type of joint is limited by the ligaments and bony processes surrounding the articulation. The carpal joints (except those of the capitate with the scaphoid and the lunate) and the tarsal joints (except that between the talus and navicular) are examples of this type of diarthrodial joint.

Spheroidal Joints.   Spheroidal joints also are called ball-and-socket joints, since they are formed by the articulation of a rounded convex surface with a cuplike cavity. The distal bone of the joint is capable of a wide variety of movements, including flexion, extension, abduction, adduction, rotation, and circumduction. The shoulder and hip joints are familiar examples of this form of articulation.

Cotylic Joints.   These joints are similar to spheroidal joints, but the articular surfaces resemble an ellipse rather than a circle. Cotylic joints, therefore, are also referred to as ellipsoid joints and are more restricted in motion than spheroidal joints, since they permit flexion, extension, abduction, adduction, and circumflexion but not axial rotation. The convex surface in a cotylic joint is somewhat longer in one direction and relatively shorter in the direction perpendicular to the long one, producing an ovoid articular surface which is received into an elliptical cavity that forms the concave surface of the joint. Cotylic joints are further subdivided according to whether they are simple or compound. *A simple cotylic joint* is one whose articular capsule encloses only one pair of articulating surfaces, while in a *compound cotylic joint* the articular capsule encloses more than one pair of articulating surfaces. The metacarpophalangeal joints of the hand are examples of simple cotylic joints, and the radiocarpal (wrist) joint is an example of a compound cotylic joint.

Hinge Joints. These joints permit motion in only one plane, flexion and extension. A hinge joint is described also as a "ginglymus." The articular surfaces of this type of joint are joined together by strong collateral ligaments that restrict lateral movement, but the extent of flexion and extension in the joint may be considerable. The best examples of hinge joints are the interphalangeal joints of the hand and foot and the humero-ulnar (elbow) joint. In these joints the range of flexion exceeds that of extension, but extension is considered to occur when the flexed joint is returned to its resting position.

Condylar Joints. In condylar joints one bone articulates with the other by two distinct articular surfaces whose movements are not dissociable. Each of these articular surfaces is referred to as a condyle. Either the convex or concave surface of the joint may be termed a "condyle"; thus the knee has tibial condyles as well as femoral condyles. Condylar joints resemble hinge joints in their movements but differ from them in the structure of their articular surfaces. The articular condyles of this type of joint may be close together and enclosed in the same articular capsule, as in the knee, or they may be widely separated and enclosed in separate articular capsules, as in the paired temporomandibular joints.

Trochoid or Pivot Joints In trochoid or pivot joints the movement of the joint is limited to rotation. This type of joint is formed by a bony pivotlike process turning within a ring or by a ring turning around a bony pivot. The ring portion of the joint is formed partly by bone and partly by a fibrous ligament. The proximal radio-ulnar joint is a trochoid joint in which the radial head rotates within the ring formed by the radial notch of the ulna and the annular ligament. The atlanto-odontal joint (medial atlanto-axial joint) is an example of a trochoid joint in which the ring, formed by the anterior arch and transverse ligament of the atlas, rotates around the odontoid process of the axis.

Sellar Joints. These have saddle-shaped articular surfaces. In this form of joint, a convex surface articulates with a concave surface in such a manner as to allow flexion, extension, abduction, adduction, and circumduction, but no axial rotation. The classic example of a sellar joint is the carpometacarpal joint of the thumb.

Systematic Method of Examination

A systematic method of examining joints is the quickest and easiest way of obtaining the available information. The examiner often begins with the joints of the upper extremity and proceeds to the joints of the trunk and the lower extremity, but the reverse of this procedure is just as effective and is preferred on some occasions. In either instance corresponding paired joints are compared systematically with each other and with respect to normalcy or abnormality for the particular joint. Inspection and palpation supplement each other; they usually can be performed together and can be followed by evaluation of joint motion.

The patient should be as comfortable as possible. Since muscles and tendons overlie and surround most joints, they must be as soft and relaxed as possible if the physician is to examine the underlying joint adequately and obtain an accurate assessment of the status of the joint. Rough or forceful handling of inflamed joints may cause not only severe pain but also muscle spasm and loss of patient cooperation so that further examination becomes difficult or unreliable. Excessive muscle spasm and guarding can usually be avoided by firm support of the area being examined and gentle handling of painful joint areas. When the examination of a painful joint requires moving it from the neutral and relaxed position, care should be taken to return the extremity slowly to a comfortable position before withdrawing the examiner's support; quick motions should be avoided. When examining tendons, the examiner must be anatomically accurate and certain that the tendon and not an adjacent nerve or other tissue is being palpated. A simple explanation to the patient of what is being done or is to be done during the examination is reassuring and often is necessary to obtain reliable observations.

Important Physical Signs of Arthritis

"Arthritis" is a general term used to describe the existence of disease *within* the joint itself. Since a typical diarthrodial joint consists of subchondral bone, articular cartilage, and a synovial membrane, one or more of these structures must be affected to permit accurate use of the term "arthritis." Synovitis, or inflammation of the synovial membrane, from whatever cause, is therefore synonymous with arthritis, although arthritis by definition may also include involvement of the articular cartilage or subchondral bone or both, with or without synovitis. However, the presence or absence of synovitis is often the most accessible and therefore the most important physical finding in the detection of arthritis. Either thickening of the synovial membrane or articular effusion is indicative of synovitis, and often both are present simultaneously in the same joint. The most common signs of articular synovitis are swelling, tenderness, and limitation of motion.

Swelling.   Swelling about a joint may be caused by intra-articular effusion, synovial thickening, periarticular soft-tissue inflammation such as bursitis or tendinitis, bony enlargement, or extra-articular fat pads. These conditions need to be differentiated from one another. Soft-tissue swelling may be either intra-articular or extra-articular in origin. It is particularly important to differentiate intra-articular soft-tissue swelling from extra-articular or periarticular involvement, since intra-articular soft-tissue swelling is indicative of arthritis (synovitis). The term "joint enlargement" is a generalization which should be avoided, as it does not distinguish joint swelling, periarticular swelling, and bony enlargement. Although muscle atrophy makes synovial effusions relatively more evident, it also may give a misleading impression of bony enlargement of a joint.

The synovial membrane is the "soft tissue" of the joint and is commonly inflamed, infected, irritated, or otherwise involved early in various arthritic processes. The resulting change in the synovial membrane may be detected by careful physical examination earlier than the involvement of other affected, hard, articular structures. Although synovial thickening and effusion are frequently associated, the examiner should try to recognize the extent of each even though this is not always possible.

Familiarity with the anatomic configuration of the synovial membrane in various joints aids in differentiating the soft-tissue swelling due to synovitis (articular effusion or synovial thickening) from the swelling of periarticular tissues. On physical examination the presence of an effusion of a joint ("joint fluid") is often demonstrated by a visible or a palpable bulging of the joint capsule or by both. Since the synovial fluid lies in a closed sac, compression of one portion of this sac causes the fluid to shift within the sac and adds to the distention of the sac elsewhere. A thickened synovial membrane with or without palpable effusion indicates arthritis (synovitis), and palpable fluid in the joint generally indicates arthritis (synovitis) even though the synovial membrane may not be palpably thickened. The normal synovial membrane is not palpable, whereas the thickened or abnormal synovial membrane may have a "doughy" or "boggy" consistency on palpation. In some joints the margin of the synovial membrane can be delineated on physical examination by compressing synovial fluid into one of the extreme limits of its reflection. The edge of the resulting bulge thus may be palpated more easily and represents a summation of the synovial membrane and the movable fluid within the synovial cavity. If this palpable edge is within the anatomic confines of the synovial membrane and disappears on release of the compression, the distention may be regarded as representing synovial effusion; if it persists, it is indicative of a thickened synovial membrane. However, reliable differentiation between synovial thickening and effusion is not always possible by physical examination. There is a small amount of synovial fluid present in a normal joint, but it is not palpable; palpable fluid in a joint is abnormal and nearly always indicates synovitis. Occasionally, intrasynovial objects, such as loose bodies, "rice bodies," or fibrin clots, may be palpated.

The examiner should be able to determine by palpation and inspection whether or not a patient has joint swelling. The presence of swelling is a definite and significant finding; therefore, terms such as "questionable swelling" and "possible swelling" used to conceal uncertainty should be avoided. However, when it is difficult to make a decision from physical examination about the presence of early or minimal swelling, repetition of the examination and experience with accurate examination of joints will aid in the determination of whether synovitis is present or not.

Tenderness. Localization of tenderness by palpation should make it apparent whether the reaction is intra-articular or in periarticular structures such as fat pads, tendon attachments, ligaments, bursae, muscles, or skin. Because tenderness is at least partly a subjective reaction, the degree of tenderness should be correlated with the emotional state of the patient. Proper interpretation of the presence of tenderness on palpation requires adequate relaxation of the muscles and tendons in the area being examined. Excessive muscle spasm may make reliable evaluation of tenderness difficult or impossible.

When possible, the examiner should try to differentiate between the pain due to distention of the synovial membrane and the pain caused by a localized inflammatory process in soft tissues. This can usually be done during the physical examination by careful localization of tender areas to specific anatomic structures. Bursal pain with or without tenderness, for example, is elicited only by motions that disturb the bursa, whereas in joint (synovial) tenderness or pain and inflammation all motions of the affected joint cause pain. Recognition of the localization of inflammatory processes in either the synovial membrane or the perisynovial tissues or both is important because, in the course of certain rheumatic diseases such as episodic rheumatoid arthritis, gout, acute rheumatic fever, palindromic rheumatism, and lupus erythematosus, inflammatory perisynovial or extra-articular reactions may be more significant or may be an earlier finding than synovial distention.

Range of Motion. The range as well as the type of motion in a normal joint depends on the shape of the articular surfaces (as described earlier in this chapter), the restraining effect of supporting ligaments, and the control exerted by muscles acting on the joint. Since limitation of motion is a common manifestation of articular disease, it is important to know the normal type and range of motion in order to detect limitation of motion resulting from abnormalities of the joint or adjacent structures. In subsequent chapters, the type and range of motion normally present in each joint are described, but generally the emphasis in the text will be on limitation of motion because of its importance and significance as a physical finding on examination of joints.

Limitation of motion may occur on either active or passive motion. In the former instance, motion is restricted when the patient attempts voluntary movement of a part; in the latter, motion is restricted when the examiner attempts movement of a part with the patient's muscles relaxed. When the active and passive ranges of motion are not equal, the passive range is usually greater and is thus the more reliable indication of the actual range of motion. However, whenever possible the active range of motion should be observed before the passive range of motion is determined. To some extent, information with regard to active range of motion becomes evident from the history (see p. 18), including a detailed description of the activities of daily living. This information is supplemented by observations made during physical examination. Discrepancies between active and passive ranges of motion may give valuable clues to abnormalities of the joints. A patient may restrict the range of passive motion if he fears that the examiner may hurt him and thus may actually have a greater range of active motion. On the other hand, he may not be able to move a joint fully because of pain from one or another of the tissues used mechanically to produce specific motions (for example, from swollen bursae, nodular tendon sheaths, torn or ruptured tendons, or otherwise affected tendons, tendon sheaths, or tendinous attachments) or because of muscle weakness or misuse of antagonist muscles. Yet with careful examination in these instances the range of passive motion may be nearly normal. Normally the ranges of active and of passive motion should be approximately the same when only intra-articular disease is present

Limitation of joint motion may be transient or permanent. Transient (reversible) limitation of motion may be due to (1) muscle spasm from fear or pain, (2) periarticular stiffness that improves with repeated movements, (3) intra-articular effusion and synovitis, (4) "locking" secondary to loose bodies in a joint, defects or disorders of the meniscus, or malposition of tendons, and (5) fibrous proliferation producing intra-articular or periarticular adhesions, tenosynovitis, or contractures of muscles, fasciae, and tendons. Permanent limitation of motion may be due to intra-articular or extra-articular causes. The former include fibrous or bony ankylosis, destruction of articular surfaces, subluxation, or impingement of bony spurs. Extra-articular causes may be tightening of the articular capsule or tendinous and fascial contractures.

Other Important Physical Signs. These include temperature and color changes in the skin over a joint, crepitation, and deformity. *Changes in temperature and color* can best be interpreted by comparison with the opposite joint. Increase in warmth and redness of the skin is a variable finding, which may or may not be apparent in the presence of articular synovitis.

Crepitation is a palpable or audible grating or crunching sensation produced by motion. It may or may not be accompanied by discomfort. Crepitation occurs when roughened articular or extra-articular surfaces are rubbed together, either by active motion or by manual compression in the course of examination. Fine crepitation is often palpable over joints involved by a chronic inflammatory arthritis, such as rheumatoid arthritis, and usually indicates roughening of the opposing cartilage surfaces as a result of erosion or the formation of granulation tissue. Coarse crepitation is also due to irregularity of the cartilage surfaces caused by either inflammatory or noninflammatory arthritis, but it is more common in the latter condition. Crepitation from within the joint should be differentiated from cracking sounds caused by the slipping of ligaments or tendons over bony surfaces during motion. The latter usually are of less significance to the diagnosis of joint disease and may be heard over many normal joints. In scleroderma a peculiar coarse, creaking, leathery crepitation may be palpable or audible about the knees, wrists, and other joints. This crepitus is produced by a rubbing together of the roughened surfaces of articular membranes or periarticular tendons and tendon sheaths.

Deformity may occur as bony enlargement, articular subluxation, contracture, and ankylosis in abnormal positions.

The application and interpretation of these physical signs as they relate more specifically to the various joints will be described in later chapters.

MUSCLE TESTING

Muscle tests are used to determine the presence, extent, and degree of muscle weakness resulting from diseases, injury, or disuse. Muscle function and joint function are closely related; that is, the use of muscles is influenced by the status of the joints moved by those muscles and vice versa. Therefore, interpretation of the results of testing the function of one of these systems often depends on knowledge of the condition of the other.

Because of the great variability of muscle strength among different people and the requirement of full cooperation by the patient during testing, the accurate judging of muscle strength in the clinical setting can be difficult. Many systems have been described for grading muscle strength. One common and useful method employing numerals includes six grades, 5 through 0. Grade 5 indicates 100 per cent strength (normal) with complete range of motion against gravity with full resistance. Grade 4 indicates 75 per cent strength (good) with complete range of motion against gravity with some resistance. Grade 3 indicates 50 per cent strength (fair) with complete range of motion against gravity. Grade 2 indicates 25 per cent strength (poor) with complete range of motion with gravity eliminated. Grade 1 indicates 10 per cent strength (trace) with evidence of slight muscle contractility (visible or by palpation) but no joint motion. Grade 0 indicates 0 per cent strength with no evidence of contractility. When testing muscles of poor strength, the portion of the body being evaluated should be supported or positioned properly to eliminate the effect of gravity. For example, instead of testing flexion of the hip while the patient sits with legs hanging over the edge of the table, the patient can be evaluated while lying on his side with the weight of the legs supported by the table during attempts to flex the hip. The palpation of muscle bellies and tendons during muscle contraction is often helpful in determining the status and function of specific muscles.

Muscle function can be assessed with the patient in a number of positions, but grading muscle strength is accomplished best by the use of positions to be described in later chapters. If the muscles being tested move a joint that has impaired function secondary to synovitis or to some other articular cause, evaluation of muscle strength may have to be carried out with very little joint motion or even isometrically.

Techniques of muscle testing are described in subsequent chapters in relation to the particular joint or joints with which the functions of the muscle are most closely integrated. The muscles that are most important in the various joint motions (the prime movers) are listed. Also given (when recognized) are the muscles that may assist in portions of these motions or that function under certain circumstances (the accessory muscles). The peripheral nerve and spinal root supply to the muscles that are the prime movers of the various motions are indicated parenthetically.

In the descriptions of muscle testing the examiner is instructed to stabilize the portion of the limb or trunk proximal to the joint being moved. It should be appreciated that this portion usually cannot be immobilized completely but should be held in as stable a position as possible. Selected illustrations to aid in the performance of muscle tests are included in each chapter. For more detailed information the reader is referred to the suggested reading at the end of this chapter.

THE JOINT CHART

Purpose and Essential Features

A permanent record of examinations of the joints is of particular help in determining progress of arthritic disease. A satisfactory chart for recording observations made during examination of the joints and also for prompting the examiner to make a complete record (1) provides the necessary completeness, (2) is convenient, and (3) is adaptable for use by different examiners. It contains space for a complete description of swelling, tenderness, and limitation of motion of each joint whether normal or abnormal and for other important articular or periarticular findings. Such a chart is especially useful for the systematic recording of information obtained in research or investigative studies of patients whose long-term course must be followed closely. A more abbreviated chart indicating and recording only abnormal findings may be satisfactory for other requirements. A generally satisfactory detailed chart is illustrated in Table 2–1. A shorter method of recording these data will be described also.

Method

Abbreviations. To avoid a cumbersome chart, abbreviations are necessary. Abbreviations for the names of joints that are used in the chart are as follows: temporomandibular (T-M), sternoclavicular (S-C),

TABLE 2-1. EXAMPLE OF CHART FOR RECORDING
JOINT EXAMINATION*

Name _____ Date _____

Joint	Right (Rt.)				Left (Lt.)			
	S	T	L	COMMENTS	S	T	L	COMMENTS
T-M	0	0	0		0	0	0	
S-C	0	0	0		0	0	0	
M-S†	0	0	0					
A-C	0	0	0		0	0	0	
Sh	0	2		Abd. 60° (or grade 1+)	0	0	0	
				Ext. rot. 60° (or grade 1+)				
				Int. rot. 60° (or grade 1+)				
Elb	0	0	0		0	0	0	
Wr	1+	1−		Dorsiflexion 35° (or grade 2)	0	0	0	
MCP	0	0	0 ⎫		MCP$_2$ 1	1−	0 ⎫	
PIP	0	0	0 ⎬ Fist 100%		PIP$_2$ 1+	0	0 ⎬ Fist 100%	
DIP	0	0	0 ⎭		0	0	0 ⎭	
Hip	0	0	0		0	0	0	
Kn	1	1		Ext. 15° (or grade 1)	0	0	0	
				Flex. 115° (or grade 1)				
Ank	0	0	0		0	0	0	
S-T	0	0	0		0	0	0	
MTP	0	0	0		MTP$_2$ 1	1	0	
PIP	0	0	0		0	0	0	
DIP	0	0	0		0	0	0	

Spine
    Cervical
        Atlas (vertebrae 1 & 2) T_0 L_0
        Vertebrae 3–7 T_0 L_0
    Thoracic
        Costochondral T_0 L_0
        Chest expansion   12.5 cm
    Lumbar T_0 L_0
        Lumbosacral T_0 L_0
    Sacroiliac T_0
    Coccyx T_0
Posture—Mild upper thoracic rounding
Gait—Normal
                    Examiner _____

*For explanation of abbreviations, see text.
†The manubriosternal joint is an unpaired joint, but it is listed with joints of the
right side for convenience.

manubriosternal (M-S), costochondral (C-C), acromioclavicular (A-C),
shoulder (Sh), elbow (Elb), wrist (Wr), metacarpophalangeal (MCP),
proximal interphalangeal (PIP), distal interphalangeal (DIP), hip (no abbreviation necessary), knee (Kn), ankle (Ank), subtalar (S-T), and metatarsophalangeal (MTP), respectively. Other appropriate abbreviations,
such as S-I for sacroiliac, may be used if desired. The digits are num-
bered 1 through 5 starting with the thumb in the case of the hand and
with the great toe of the foot. Some orthopedic surgeons prefer to designate individual fingers by description rather than by the numbering of 1

through 5 as follows: thumb, index finger, middle finger, ring finger, and little finger.

In recording the degree of swelling (S), tenderness (T), and limitation of motion (L) of a joint, a quantitative estimate of gradation based on a system of grades from 0 to 4 is convenient and may be used as follows: 0 means normal; 1, mildly abnormal; 2, moderately abnormal; 3, markedly abnormal; and 4, maximally abnormal. This grading is used in Table 2–1.

The abbreviation S as used in the chart refers to synovial swelling, thickening, or effusion, or combinations thereof. If extra-articular edema or capsular, bursal, or osseous enlargement is present, a specific description of this is needed to avoid confusion in the use of the abbreviation S as the indicator for synovial swelling. Synovial swelling is best evaluated by the simultaneous use of both inspection and palpation. Swelling of grade 1 severity, designated in the chart in Table 2–1 as "1" in the column "S" and conveniently referred to as "S_1," may not be apparent on casual inspection but should be recognizable to an experienced examiner. Swelling of grades 2, 3, and 4 severity (S_2, S_3, and S_4, respectively) indicates increasing degrees of visible distention or thickening of the synovial membrane. Swelling of grade 1 or 2 is much more frequently observed than swelling of grade 3 or 4; swelling of grade 4 is actually rare. Because swelling of grade 1 or 2 occurs frequently, some examiners prefer to use divisions within these grades, such as $1-$, $1+$, $2-$ and $2+$, conveniently referred to as S_{1-}, S_{1+}, S_{2-}, S_{2+}, to indicate variations which can be observed rather than to use grades 3 and 4 when these extremes of swelling are not precisely justified. Since the synovial membrane (and articular capsule) is generally less capable of marked distention when swelling occurs acutely than when swelling develops chronically, the extreme degrees of synovial swelling are more often found when the synovitis has developed slowly or been present chronically. In individual instances the degree of swelling may be the same as, or disproportionately greater or lesser than, the amount of tenderness. The grade of swelling and the grade of tenderness (see following) are coexisting indicators of articular abnormalities but need to be evaluated separately.

Tenderness of the synovial membranes or perisynovial capsule or both is generally indicated by T. Tenderness of other structures needs to be specifically differentiated and designated accordingly (for example, tendons, fat pads, and semilunar cartilages). Tenderness of grade 1 severity (T_1) indicates slight or mild tolerable discomfort on palpation. Grade 2 tenderness (T_2) indicates more severe pain on ordinary palpation which the patient prefers not to tolerate. Grade 3 tenderness (T_3) describes marked and more intolerable pain with even light palpation or pressure. Grade 4 tenderness (T_4) is less commonly encountered and indicates pain which may be caused by a mild stimulus such as blowing air onto the joint, light touch, slight motion of the skin overlying the joint, or the vibration of heavy footsteps nearby. It should be noted also

whether pain is present during rest or only with movement. Some observers use + and − to denote slight variations within a grade when
describing the severity of tenderness in a joint. For example, tenderness,
grade 2 (T_2) may be used to indicate pain on palpation which the patient
prefers not to tolerate but from which he does not pull away involuntarily, whereas T_{2+} is indicative of pain from which the patient involuntarily withdraws the examined joint, but the pain is still less than that
graded as 3.

In the case of *limitation of motion* (L), grade 1 may be used to
indicate about 25 per cent loss of motion; grade 2, about 50 per cent;
grade 3, about 75 per cent; and grade 4, 100 per cent or complete ankylosis. Again the symbols + and − may be used to denote variations
within a grade; thus, a 35 per cent loss of motion would equal grade 1+
and an 85 per cent loss of motion would equal grade 3+. The range of
motion of the joints in degrees may be recorded in addition to, or in
preference to, grading by the numerical scale and is a more accurate
recording of the motion. In order to maintain consistency and simplicity
in measuring the range of joint motion, the neutral position of a joint
has been designated as "0 degrees" ("0°" in chart) throughout the text. In
the past, some physicians have used "180 degrees" to designate the neutral position for certain joints, such as the knee and the elbow, but this is
confusing and should be avoided for the sake of uniformity or standard-
ization in recording the findings. Generally, motion in the knee, finger
joints, and elbow is suited to recording by measurement in degrees,
whereas motion in the wrist, ankle, metatarsophalangeal joints, and temporomandibular joints is evaluated more conveniently and just as satisfactorily by the use of gradations. In the shoulder and hip, abduction and
adduction are often best measured in degrees, but rotation is measured
either by degrees or by gradations.

Interpretation of the Chart (Table 2–1)

The chart in Table 2–1 indicates the presence of a moderately
tender and limited right shoulder; a mildly swollen (synovial) and tender
right wrist with moderate limitation of dorsiflexion; a slightly swollen
(synovial) and tender metacarpophalangeal joint of the left second finger;
a mildly swollen (synovial) proximal interphalangeal joint of the left second finger; a slightly swollen (synovial) and tender right knee with slight
limitation of motion in both extension and flexion; and a mildly swollen
(synovial) and tender metatarsophalangeal joint of the left second toe.

As mentioned earlier, comments describing swelling or tenderness
are often necessary for greater specificity in addition to grading. Thus,
tenderness in the shoulder might be due to involvement of the subdeltoid portion of the subacromial bursa, the bicipital extension (or outpouching) of the articular synovial membrane, the rotator cuff of the

shoulder, or the synovial membrane of the glenohumeral joint, and the specific site would have to be noted. An additional statement to interpret and record observations relative to muscular weakness, cutaneous or subcutaneous contractures, nodules, local heat and color changes, bursal or tenosynovial swelling, and tenderness of fibrous attachments should be made when any of these conditions is present.

An Abbreviated Record

If a more abbreviated record were being used, the joint examination given in detail in Table 2–1 could be recorded simply and briefly as Rt. Sh S_0, T_2, L_{1+}; Rt. Wr S_{1+}, T_{1-}, L_2; Lt. MCP_2, S_1, T_{1-}, L_0; Lt. PIP_2, S_{1+}, T_0, L_0; Rt. Kn S_1, T_1, L_1 (lacks 15° of extension); Lt. MTP_2 S_1, T_1 L_0. The omission of certain detailed and important data is avoided by using the more detailed information when indicated.

OTHER RECORDING TECHNIQUES

Other methods of evaluating and recording the status and function of the joints have been devised and may be useful in certain circum-

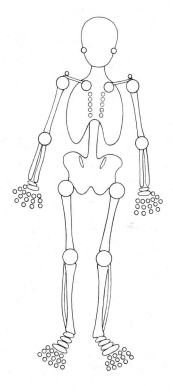

Figure 2–2. Schematic skeleton with articulations marked, which may be used to record the status of individual joints in a patient with arthritis.

stances. These methods include determining the number of clinically abnormal joints, the size of joints by using a metal tape measure or jeweler's rings, the degree of warmth by using thermography, and the amount of tenderness by using a dolorimeter. The grip strength can be measured by having a patient grasp and squeeze a partially inflated (20 mm Hg) sphygmomanometer cuff. The use of joints can be studied by determining the time required to walk 50 feet or the time required or the ability to perform other specified coordinated activities or activities of daily living (ADL).

Figure 2–2 shows a stamp modified from an initial design by Lansbury on which all involved or abnormal joints may be marked. Reference may be made to the following sources for these and other useful methods of recording the joint examination.

SUGGESTED READING FOR ADDITIONAL INFORMATION

Recording Techniques

1. American Academy of Orthopaedic Surgeons. Committee for the Study of Joint Motion: Joint Motion: Method of Measuring and Recording. Revised edition. Chicago, American Academy of Orthopaedic Surgeons, 1965, 87 pp.
2. McCarty DJ Jr: Methods of evaluating rheumatoid arthritis. In: Hollander JL, McCarty DJ Jr (editors): Arthritis and Allied Conditions: A Textbook of Rheumatology. Eighth edition. Philadelphia, Lea & Febiger, 1972, pp. 419–438.
3. Rusk HA: Rehabilitation Medicine. Fourth edition. St. Louis, CV Mosby Company, 1977, pp. 140–153.
4. Kottke FJ: Training for functional independence. In: Krusen FH, Kottke FJ, Ellwood PM Jr: Handbook of Physical Medicine and Rehabilitation. Second edition. Philadelphia, WB Saunders Company, 1971, pp. 473–487.

General Rheumatology

1. Rodnan GP, McEwen CW, Wallace SL (editors): Primer on the rheumatic diseases. JAMA 224(suppl 5):1–152, 1973.
2. Hollander JL, McCarty DJ Jr. (editors): Arthritis and Allied Conditions: A Textbook of Rheumatology. Eighth edition. Philadelphia, Lea & Febiger, 1972, 1593 pp.
3. Boyle JA, Buchanan WW: Clinical Rheumatology. Philadelphia, FA Davis Company, 1971, 587 pp.
4. Gardner DL: The Pathology of Rheumatoid Arthritis. Baltimore, Williams & Wilkins Company, 1972, 259 pp.
5. Rusk HA: Rehabilitation Medicine. Fourth edition. St. Louis, CV Mosby Company, 1977, 675 pp. (especially Chapters 7, 8, 9, and 20).
6. McKusick VA: Heritable Disorders of Connective Tissue. Fourth edition. St. Louis, CV Mosby Company, 1972, 878 pp.
7. Kendall HO, Kendall FP, Wadsworth GE: Muscles, Testing and Function. Second edition. Baltimore, Williams & Wilkins Company, 1971, 284 pp.
8. Daniels L, Worthingham C: Muscle Testing: Techniques of Manual Examination. Third edition. Philadelphia, WB Saunders Company, 1972, 165 pp.

Anatomy of Joints

1. Warwick R, Williams PL: Gray's Anatomy. 35th British edition. Philadelphia, WB Saunders Company, 1973, 1471 pp.
2. Romanes GJ (editor): Cunningham's Textbook of Anatomy. 11th edition. London, Oxford University Press, 1972, 996 pp.

3. Goss CM (editor): Gray's Anatomy of the Human Body. 29th American edition. Philadelphia, Lea & Febiger, 1973, 1466 pp.
4. Anson BJ, McVay CB: Surgical Anatomy. Fifth edition. Philadelphia, WB Saunders Company, 1971, 1241 pp. Vols. I and II (especially Vol. II, pp. 725–1241).
5. Hollinshead WH: Anatomy for Surgeons. Second edition. New York, Harper Medical Division, Harper and Row. Vol. 1, 1968, 619 pp. (especially the chapter on the cricoarytenoid joint). Vol. 3, 1969, 894 pp. (especially chapters on the acromioclavicular joint, shoulder, elbow, spine, hip, knee, and ankle and foot).
6. Barnett CH, Davies DV, MacConaill MA: Synovial Joints: Their Structure and Mechanics. Springfield, Ill., Charles C Thomas, 1961, 304 pp.

chapter **3**

The Temporomandibular Joint

ESSENTIAL ANATOMY

INSPECTION

PALPATION

MOVEMENT AND RANGE OF MOTION

MUSCLE TESTING

ESSENTIAL ANATOMY

The temporomandibular joint is formed by the fossa and the articular tubercle of the temporal bone and the condyle of the mandible. An articular disk of fibrocartilage divides the joint into two cavities each lined with synovial membrane. The synovial membrane is covered by a loose fibrous capsule which is strengthened laterally by the temporomandibular ligament. The paired temporomandibular joints are classified as a condylar joint, since one bone (the mandible) articulates with the other (the skull) by two distinct articular surfaces or condyles. Thus, each temporomandibular joint represents a condyle of the condylar joint, even though they are widely separated and are enclosed by different articular capsules (Fig. 3–1).

INSPECTION

Swelling in this joint must be moderate or marked before it is apparent on inspection. If swelling is detectable, it appears as a rounded bulge in the area overlying the joint just anterior to the external auditory meatus (Fig. 3–2). Arthritis of the temporomandibular joint in young in-

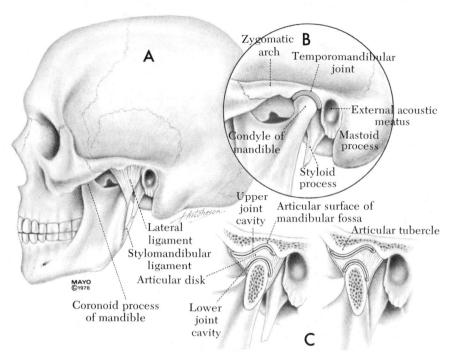

Zygomatic arch
B
Temporomandibular joint
External acoustic meatus
Condyle of mandible
Mastoid process
Styloid process
Upper joint cavity
Articular surface of mandibular fossa
Articular tubercle
Lateral ligament
Stylomandibular ligament
Articular disk
A
Coronoid process of mandible
Lower joint cavity
C

Figure 3–1. The temporomandibular joint. *A.* Lateral aspect of skull showing the relationship of the temporomandibular joint and mandible to neighboring structures. The lateral ligament covers and strengthens the lateral aspect of the joint capsule. *B.* Diagram showing the relationship of the temporomandibular joint to the external acoustic canal and zygomatic arch. Synovial membrane is shown in blue. *C.* Sagittal section of the temporomandibular joint illustrating the relationship of synovial membranes (shown in blue) and the intra-articular disk. With the jaw closed, on the left, the head of the condyle of the mandible and the articular disk lie within the mandibular fossa. With the jaw open, on the right, the condyle turns in a hinge fashion on the disk and both glide forward within the joint capsule.

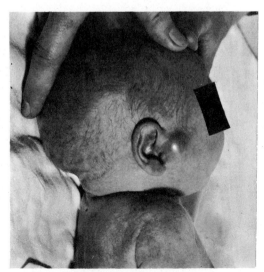

Figure 3–2. Acute septic involvement of the temporomandibular joint due to staphylococcal infection in an infant.

dividuals may result in a disturbance of bone growth characterized by a shortened lower jaw (micrognathia; Fig. 3–3).

PALPATION

The joint can be located by placing the tip of the forefinger just anterior to the external auditory meatus and asking the patient to open his mouth. The tip of the examiner's finger then drops into an area overlying the joint proper. Moderate degrees of swelling in the joint prevent the fingertip from entering the depressed area overlying the joint. Swelling of marked degree may be palpable as a rounded, often fluctuant mass overlying the temporomandibular joint. By palpating the condyle and noting its location in the mandibular fossa with the patient's jaw closed, partially open, and wide open, the physician can determine various degrees of dislocation. Palpable or audible snapping or clicking of the temporomandibular joint occurs in many people without evidence of arthritic disease. In the presence of palpable synovitis, local tenderness and warmth may be noted on palpation of the temporomandibular joint.

MOVEMENT AND RANGE OF MOTION

The temporomandibular joint permits three types of motion: opening and closing of the jaws, protrusion and retrusion of the mandible (anterior and posterior motion), and lateral or side-to-side motion.

Movement at each temporomandibular joint has two components. The inferior portion of the joint is formed by the mandibular condyle and articular disk and functions as a hinge joint, whereas the superior portion of the joint between the temporal bone and articular disk acts as a sliding joint, allowing both the disk and the mandible to glide forward, backward, and from side to side. When the jaws are opened and closed, motion, causing the mandible to rotate about a center of suspension slightly above the angle of the mandible, occurs in both portions of each joint. Anteroposterior movements of the mandible are performed mainly by the gliding action of the superior compartments, and lateral displacement of the jaw causes one articular disk to glide forward while the other remains in position. The grinding movements of chewing are produced by alternate movements in both compartments.

Vertical motion in this joint is determined most readily by measuring the space between the upper and lower incisor teeth with the patient's mouth open maximally. Care should be taken to keep the lower jaw somewhat protruded during this measurement, since maximal opening of the mandible depends on adequate forward positioning of the lower jaw as well as on the degree of vertical motion. Normally, this distance will be about 3 to 6 cm (Fig. 3–4). Lateral motion of the jaw is

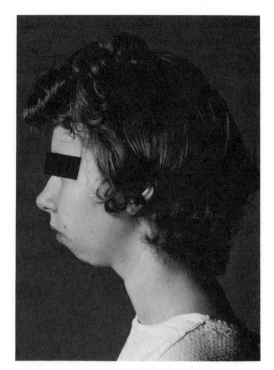

Figure 3–3. Receding chin and underslung jaw (micrognathia) in a patient with juvenile rheumatoid arthritis involving the temporomandibular joint.

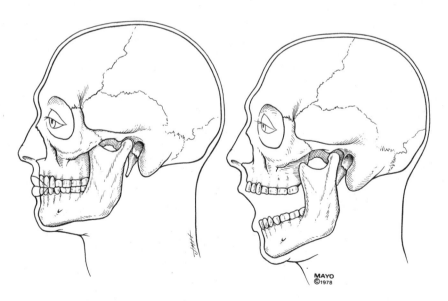

Figure 3–4. Schematic drawing showing the range of motion of temporomandibular joint. The condyle of the mandible glides forward as the jaw is depressed.

measured by having the patient partially open his mouth, protrude the lower jaw, and then move the lower jaw from side to side. Since the position of the mandible in the anteroposterior direction can cause considerable variation in the degree of lateral motion of the jaw, it is best to evaluate lateral motion with the jaw protruded as far as possible (Fig. 3–5). The extent of lateral motion of the lower jaw is normally about 1 or 2 cm. Lateral motion may be lost earlier and to a greater degree than vertical motion. Finally, the patient is asked to protrude the lower jaw to see if it deviates to one side during protrusion.

MUSCLE TESTING

The muscles that close the mandible on the maxilla are the temporalis (deep temporal branches of the mandibular division of the facial nerve, C7), the masseter (masseteric nerve from the mandibular division of the trigeminal nerve, C5), and the medial pterygoid (medial pterygoid nerve of the mandibular division of the trigeminal nerve) muscles. The muscles that open or depress the mandible are the lateral pterygoid and suprahyoid muscles. The suprahyoid muscles that assist in depressing the mandible are the digastric (mandibular division of the trigeminal nerve to the posterior belly and the facial nerve to the anterior belly), the mylo-

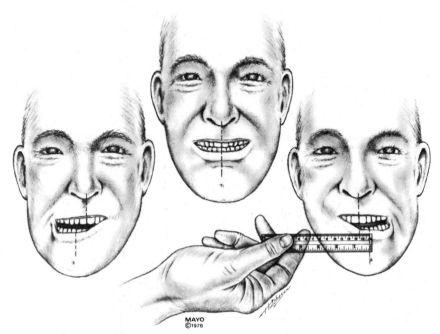

MAYO
©1978

Figure 3–5. Schematic drawing showing a method of measuring lateral movement of temporomandibular joints.

hyoid (mandibular division of the trigeminal nerve), and the geniohyoid (hypoglossal nerve, C1).

The temporalis and masseter muscles are most readily assessable. The patient is instructed to close the jaws tightly. The size, firmness, and strength of the muscles are determined and graded by the examiner, who uses his fingertips to palpate the temporalis muscles in the temporal regions of the head and the masseter muscles below the zygomatic arches on both sides of the face and then compares one side with the other. The lateral pterygoid (lateral pterygoid nerve of the mandibular division of the trigeminal nerve) and medial pterygoid muscles on the left side are tested by having the patient move the mandible forward and laterally to the right side against graded resistance of the examiner's fingers, which are placed near the front of the mandible on the right side. The pterygoid muscles are tested on the right side by having the patient move the mandible forward and laterally to the left against the graded resistance of the examiner's hand, which is placed near the front of the left side of the mandible. Depression of the mandible is tested by instructing the patient to open his mouth against the graded resistance provided by one of the examiner's hands placed under the front of the mandible.

SUGGESTED READING FOR ADDITIONAL INFORMATION

1. Shore NA: Temporomandibular Joint Dysfunction and Occlusal Equilibration. Second edition. Philadelphia, JB Lippincott Company, 1976, 376 pp.
2. Chalmers IM, Blair GS: Rheumatoid arthritis of the temporomandibular joint: A clinical and radiological study using circular tomography. Q J Med 42:367–386, 1973.
3. Yune HY, Hall JR, Hutton CE, Klatte EC: Roentgenologic diagnosis in chronic temporomandibular joint dysfunction syndrome. Am J Roentgenol Radium Ther Nucl Med 118:401–414, 1973.

chapter **4**

The Cricoarytenoid Joint

ESSENTIAL ANATOMY
INSPECTION
PALPATION
RANGE OF MOTION
SIGNIFICANCE

ESSENTIAL ANATOMY

The paired cricoarytenoid joints are small but normally very mobile diarthrodial joints that are formed by the articulation of the facet on the upper posterolateral border of the cricoid cartilage laminae with the base of the arytenoid cartilage. Each arytenoid cartilage somewhat resembles a three-sided pyramid with the base articulating and moving on the cricoid. The vocal folds (cords) are attached to the arytenoid cartilage (Fig. 4–1), and the several muscles acting on these cartilages produce the motion of the vocal cords. Two general, closely integrated types of arytenoid movement occur during normal respiration and phonation. These are (1) rotation about an essentially vertical axis and (2) medial and lateral gliding motions whereby the arytenoid cartilages alternately approach each other and then separate. Medial rotation and medial gliding cause the vocal folds to approach each other in the course of phonation, and lateral rotation and lateral gliding separate the vocal folds during normal respiratory inspiration.

INSPECTION

The cricoarytenoid joints are viewed most conveniently by indirect laryngoscopy (mirror examination of the larynx) or by direct laryn-

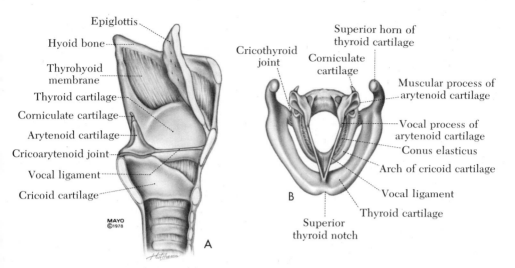

Figure 4–1. The cricoarytenoid joint of the larynx. *A.* Sagittal section. *B.* Superior view. Synovial membrane is shown in blue.

goscopy. Abnormalities that can often be seen include edema and redness about the cricoarytenoid joint and surrounding structures and varying degrees of displacement of the arytenoid cartilage. Edema and redness are associated with acute or subacute arthritis and may not be seen in more chronic phases of the disease. Scarring or roughening of the mucosa over the arytenoids may be noted in chronic arthritis. Complete displacement of the arytenoid cartilage follows severe or chronic involvement of the cricoarytenoid joint.

PALPATION

Pain resulting from pressure over the anterior aspect of the larynx or from compression of the superior cornua of the thyroid cartilage is a positive sign of cricoarytenoid arthritis. A thrill may be palpable externally over the tracheal cartilages in the neck below the thyroid cartilage. This corresponds to stridor (in patients with severe disease) and bilateral fixation of the arytenoid cartilages in the position of adduction.

Manipulation of the arytenoid cartilages with a laryngeal spatula causes pain to patients with acute cricoarytenoid arthritis.

RANGE OF MOTION

Mobility of the arytenoid cartilages can be tested by asking the patient to attempt phonation during laryngoscopy; or the examiner can try to move the cartilages or vocal cords with a laryngeal spatula. With severe or chronic arthritic involvement, fixation of the cricoarytenoid joints occurs, and attempts to separate the vocal cords are unsuccessful. This observation differentiates articular involvement from bilateral paralysis of the vocal cords.

SIGNIFICANCE

Arthritis of the cricoarytenoid joint is recognized relatively infrequently, but it is found in some patients with rheumatoid arthritis. Trauma and infection of this joint have been reported even less frequently, and a few individual cases of involvement by gout and systemic lupus erythematosus have been reported. In rheumatoid arthritis, cricoarytenoid arthritis is more common than is generally supposed when no routine examination is made for it and tends to be more severe when rheumatoid arthritis has been persistently inflamed for many years. In cases of rheumatoid arthritis, involvement of the joint may be unilateral or bilateral. Early symptoms include a feeling of fullness or discomfort in the throat that is aggravated by swallowing or speaking. The hoarseness may be intermittent and may be worse in the morning, concurrent with morning stiffness in other joints. Later, dysphagia, hoarseness, and stridor result; hoarseness and dyspnea are proportional to the degree of cricoarytenoid joint fixation. Significant obstruction of the airway is uncommon but has been fatal in some instances.

SUGGESTED READING FOR ADDITIONAL INFORMATION

1. Montgomery WW: Cricoarytenoid arthritis. Laryngoscope 73:801–836, 1963.
2. Friedman, BA, Rice DH: Rheumatoid nodules of the larynx. Arch Otolaryngol 101:361–363, 1975.
3. Funk D, Raymon F: Rheumatoid arthritis of the cricoarytenoid joints: An airway hazard. Anesth Analg (Cleve) 54:742–745, 1975.

chapter **5**

The Acromioclavicular
Joint

ESSENTIAL ANATOMY

INSPECTION AND PALPATION

MOVEMENT AND RANGE OF MOTION

ESSENTIAL ANATOMY

The acromioclavicular joint is a simple spheroidal joint formed by the lateral end of the clavicle and the medial margin of the acromion process of the scapula. There may or may not be a fibrocartilaginous articular disk in the joint cavity, but the joint is lined with synovial membrane. The joint is enveloped by a fibrous capsule that is strengthened by superior and inferior acromioclavicular ligaments. Often a subcutaneous bursa is located superficially over the acromioclavicular joint, but it rarely communicates with the joint cavity. (See Figs. 7–2 and 7–3, p. 63.)

INSPECTION AND PALPATION

Although the acromioclavicular joint lies near the surface, localized swelling and tenderness in this area are best determined by palpation rather than by inspection because of the close proximity of the joint to the prominence of the shoulder. First one acromioclavicular joint and then the other is palpated with the examiner's fingertips, and the joint on one side is compared with the joint on the other side. Palpation is best accomplished with the examiner in front of the patient and with the patient either sitting or standing. Localized tenderness and pain with movement confined to this area are observed more often than localized swelling and are more significant findings, since swelling in this region is difficult to localize accurately by inspection or palpation. Adduction of the patient's arm across his chest or shrugging of his shoulder may produce pain and help localize tenderness in disorders of the acromioclavicular joint.

MOVEMENT AND RANGE OF MOTION

The acromioclavicular joint enables the scapula to move vertically when the shoulder girdle rises (shrugging the shoulders) and falls. It also enables the scapula to rotate backward and forward on the clavicle. When the arm is raised above the head, the acromioclavicular joint participates in the movement of the scapula and the accompanying elevation of the shoulder. (Scapular movement accounts for most of the final 90 degrees of vertical motion when the arm is raised above the head.) However, actual measurements of the range of motion in the acromioclavicular joint are not necessary in the usual rheumatologic examination of the joint.

SUGGESTED READING FOR ADDITIONAL INFORMATION

1. Bateman JE: The Shoulder and Neck. Second edition. Philadelphia, WB Saunders Company, 1978, 850 pp.
2. Moseley HF: Shoulder Lesions. Third edition. Baltimore, Williams & Wilkins Company, 1969, 318 pp. (especially Chapters 10 and 11).
3. De Palma AF: Surgery of the Shoulder. Second edition. Philadelphia, JB Lippincott Company, 1973, 551 pp.

chapter **6**

The Sternoclavicular and Manubriosternal Joints

ESSENTIAL ANATOMY

INSPECTION AND PALPATION

MOVEMENT AND RANGE OF MOTION

ESSENTIAL ANATOMY

The medial end of the clavicle articulates with the sternum to form the sternoclavicular joint on each side of the upper end of the manubrium (Fig. 6–1). The sternoclavicular joint is a simple spheroidal joint. A fibrocartilaginous disk separates each joint into two separate cavities, the chondroclavicular and the chondrosternal. Both are lined with synovial membrane. A fibrous tissue capsule surrounds the entire joint and is strengthened by anterior and posterior sternoclavicular ligaments and the interclavicular ligament. The costoclavicular ligament, which is a dense fibrous band or membrane located just lateral to the joint capsule, unites the clavicle with the first rib.

The manubriosternal (sometimes referred to as sternomanubrial) joint is an amphiarthrodial joint or synchondrosis with hyaline cartilage covering the articulating ends of the manubrium and the body of the sternum (corpus sterni), which are joined together with an intervening fibrocartilage (Fig. 6–1). A joint cavity, with or without a lining of small oval cells resembling synovial lining cells, has been reported in more than one-third of the cases studied and is said to be more frequent in women than in men. The similarity of this articulation to the pubic symphysis has resulted in an alternate term for this joint, namely, the "symphysis sterni." The dual or hybrid character of the joint has also suggested the designation "diarthro-amphiarthrosis."

On the lateral margins of the superior part of the body of the

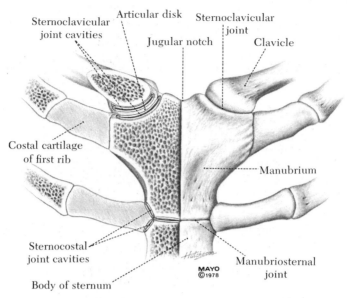

Figure 6–1. Schematic drawing of sternoclavicular, manubriosternal, and costo-sternal joints. The left side of the drawing is a frontal section view. Synovial membrane is shown in blue.

sternum are articular facets for the articulations of the second ribs (or, rarely, for the third ribs). These and the other costal articulations with the sternum are joints lined with synovial membrane, with or without intra-articular ligaments. The manubrium may fuse with the sternum some time after growth has been completed.

The junction of the manubrium and the superior part of the body of the sternum forms an obtuse sternal angle situated about 5 cm below the jugular notch on the superior border of the manubrium. This line or angle of junction has been labeled the "manubriosternal synchondrosis" and is a useful landmark or reference point for counting the ribs.

INSPECTION AND PALPATION

The sternoclavicular and manubriosternal joints lie just beneath the skin; thus, any swelling and redness in this area can easily be seen. Observing this area from an oblique angle often provides a better view than does looking at it directly, and comparison of one side with the other in this manner provides additional clarification of findings. Synovitis of the sternoclavicular joints may produce a smooth rounded swelling extending over the entire area of these joints (Fig. 6–2). With less severe synovitis the swelling may be more easily detected just lateral to the sternoclavicular joint in the depression between the clavicle and the first rib.

The chondroclavicular and chondrosternal components of the sternoclavicular joint are best palpated with the tips of the examiner's second

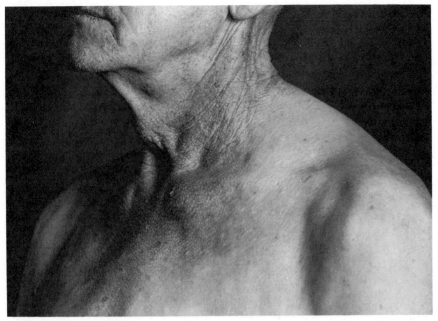

Figure 6–2. Bilateral swelling of the sternoclavicular joints in a patient with rheumatoid arthritis.

and third fingers while comparing the two sternoclavicular joints. The consistency and location of swelling and the presence or absence of tenderness and local heat can be determined easily by palpation and by such comparison.

Involvement of the manubriosternal joint is commonly overlooked clinically. Tenderness of this joint is more frequent than swelling, but there may be enough of the latter to increase the linear and horizontal prominence of the sternal angle. The joint is subject to the same articular inflammatory and destructive changes as the synovial diarthrodial joints are, especially in patients with ankylosing spondylitis or rheumatoid arthritis. In ankylosing spondylitis the involvement is similar to that of another synchondrosis, the symphysis pubis. Whether involvement of the manubriosternal joint in rheumatoid arthritis is related to the presence of a synovial or synovial-like joint lining or to a synovial membrane of the costosternal articulation of the second ribs has not been determined. Palpation and perception of local warmth, tenderness, or swelling of the manubriosternal joint are accomplished by using the tips of the examiner's fingers.

MOVEMENT AND RANGE OF MOTION

The two sternoclavicular joints are the only points of articulation of the shoulder girdle with the trunk. Thus, in any motion of the shoulder girdle there is motion of the sternoclavicular joint unless this joint is ankylosed. Discomfort may occur in the region of the sternoclavicular joint on motion of the shoulder girdle, but measurement of motion of the sternoclavicular joint in degrees is not practicable.

Motion of the manubriosternal joint is negligible, and its measurement likewise is not clinically practicable or significant.

SUGGESTED READING FOR ADDITIONAL INFORMATION

1. Laitinen H, Saksanen S, Souranta H: Involvement of the manubriosternal articulation in rheumatoid arthritis. Acta Rheum Scand 16:40–46, 1970.
2. Kormano M: A microradiographic and histological study of the manubriosternal joint in rheumatoid arthritis. Acta Rheum Scand 16:47–49, 1970.

Also refer to references at the end of Chapter 5, page 56.

chapter **7**

The Shoulder

ESSENTIAL ANATOMY

The shoulder or glenohumeral joint is a spheroidal or ball-and-socket joint formed by the articulation of the head of the humerus with the shallow glenoid cavity of the scapula (glenoid fossa). The shoulder joint allows considerable mobility of the arm and is enclosed by a group of powerful muscles and tendons that support and stabilize the joint. The joint is protected superiorly by an arch formed by the coracoid process, the acromion, and the coraco-acromial ligament. The shoulder girdle is formed by the scapula and the clavicle; they articulate with each other at the acromioclavicular joint. The main portion or body of the scapula is a large, flat, triangular bone that does not articulate with any portion of the skeleton other than the humerus and clavicle and is connected to the posterior aspect of the chest wall only by axio-appendicular muscles (Figs. 7–1 to 7–3).

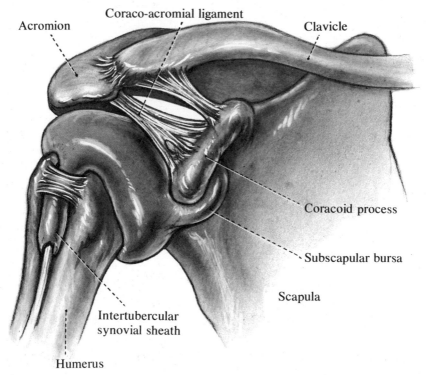

Figure 7–1. Anterior aspect of shoulder joint showing the distribution of the distended synovial membrane of the glenohumeral joint and its relationship to adjacent bony structures. Synovial membrane, bursae, and synovial sheaths in this and subsequent drawings are shown in blue unless otherwise indicated.

Articular Capsule and Synovial Membrane

The fibrous articular capsule of the shoulder completely encircles the glenohumeral joint. It is attached superiorly (proximally) to the circumference of the glenoid cavity beyond the fibrocartilaginous rim of the glenoid labrum. Inferiorly (distally), it is attached to the anatomic neck of the humerus. The articular capsule is very loose and lax and allows the bones of the joint to separate from each other. The laxity of the articular capsule permits considerable freedom of motion, which is characteristic of this joint. The articular capsule has two openings. One is an aperture in the attachment of the articular capsule to the humerus that allows the long tendon of the biceps muscle to enter the intertubercular (bicipital) groove of the humerus. The other aperture is located under the subscapular tendon and permits an extracapsular outpouching of the synovial membrane to function as a bursa for the subscapularis muscle.

The synovial membrane of the shoulder lines the inner surface of the fibrous articular capsule and also the structures that penetrate the capsule. The synovial membrane has two outpouchings, one of which

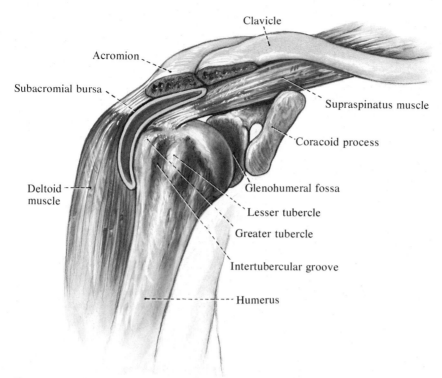

Figure 7–2. Anterior aspect of the shoulder joint showing palpable landmarks and their relationship to the subacromial bursa.

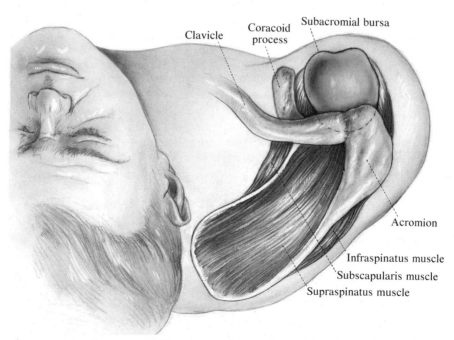

Figure 7–3. The shoulder (glenohumeral) joint viewed from above, showing bony landmarks and their relationship to the subacromial bursa.

(the subscapular portion) is actually extracapsular and functions as a bursa for the subscapularis muscle, as mentioned. The other (the bicipital portion) extends along the intertubercular (bicipital) groove on the anterior aspect of the humerus and functions as a sheath for the tendon of the long head of the biceps muscle (Fig. 7–1).

The Rotator Cuff of the Shoulder

The broad, flat tendons of the supraspinatus, infraspinatus, and teres minor muscles insert into the greater tubercle of the humerus, and the tendon of the subscapularis muscle inserts into the lesser tubercle. Together these four muscles and tendons are termed the "rotator cuff of the shoulder." The supraspinatus muscle functions primarily as an upward rotator (abductor), the infraspinatus and teres minor muscles as lateral rotators, and the subscapularis muscle as a medial rotator. Prior to their insertions, each of the four tendons is incorporated in the fibrous cylindrical capsule that encloses the shoulder joint; consequently, the articular capsule is reinforced by these tendons. Reinforcement of the capsule is accomplished anteriorly by the subscapularis tendon, superiorly by the supraspinatus tendon, and posteriorly by the infraspinatus and the teres minor tendons.

Bursae

Overlying the tendinous and capsular cuff of the shoulder is the large *subacromial bursa* (Figs. 7–2 and 7–3). The lateral extension of this bursa is termed the "subdeltoid bursa," since it lies beneath the deltoid muscle. The subacromial bursa facilitates movement of the greater tubercle of the humerus beneath the acromion during abduction of the arm. Abduction of the shoulder compresses this bursa and also causes the acromion to impinge on the insertion of the supraspinatus tendon (Fig. 7–4). The subacromial bursa communicates with the joint cavity in approximately 20 to 33 per cent of individuals past middle age. Since the supraspinatus tendon forms the roof of the shoulder capsule and the floor of the subacromial bursa (Fig. 7–2), any tear of the tendon is likely to result in a communication between the bursa and the joint cavity.

The *subcoracoid bursa* lies between the capsule of the shoulder and the coracoid process. It may be separate from, or may communicate with, the subacromial bursa. Another small bursa, called the "subcutaneous acromial bursa," lies over the acromion process. Several other bursae occur about the shoulder; these may be significant anatomically but are relatively insignificant clinically.

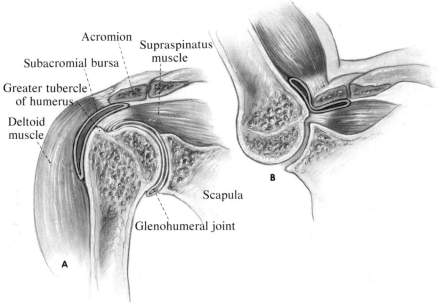

Figure 7–4. Relationship of subacromial bursa (shown in blue) to supraspinatus muscle and acromion process. *A.* In position of adduction of humerus. In order to show this bursa more clearly, the synovial membrane of the glenohumeral joint is not shown in blue. *B.* In position of abduction of humerus, the acromion impinges on the subacromial bursa and the insertion of the supraspinatus tendon.

INSPECTION

Inspection of the shoulders is performed with the patient's clothing removed to the level of the waist and, if possible, with the patient either sitting or standing. Both shoulders are compared anteriorly and posteriorly for evidence of swelling and muscular atrophy or fasciculations over the trapezius, deltoid, scapular, and pectoral muscles. Atrophy of the supraspinatus and infraspinatus muscles is recognized as a lack of fullness in the respective superior and inferior scapular fossae (Fig. 7–5). Inequality or malposition of normal bony landmarks, such as the clavicle, acromion, coracoid process, or greater tubercle of the humerus, should be apparent by comparison of both sides. If the shoulder is dislocated anteriorly, the rounded lateral aspect of the shoulder is lost and appears flattened. Posterior dislocation of the shoulder, which is relatively rare, causes a flattening of the anterior aspect of the shoulder and sometimes produces a prominence of the humeral head, which can be seen over the posterior aspect of the shoulder in a thin individual.

A moderate to considerable amount of synovitis or fluid must be present in the glenohumeral joint to cause visible distention of the articular capsule. When present, this distention usually occurs over the anterior aspect of the joint (Fig. 7–6). Occasionally, an intra-articular effusion

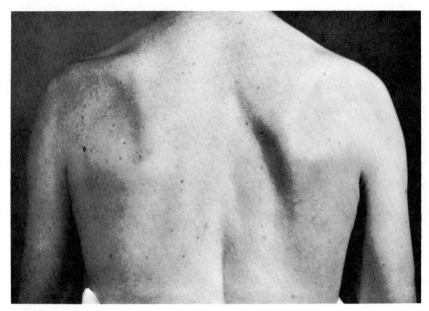

Figure 7–5. Prominence of scapulae and atrophy of scapular, rhomboid, and serratus muscles in a patient with cervical radiculitis. Scapula is more prominent on the right, but the muscular atrophy is greater on the left side.

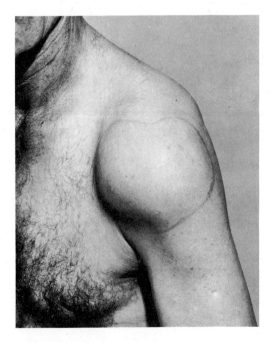

Figure 7–6. Synovial cyst of left shoulder joint of patient with rheumatoid arthritis. The fluctuant, palpable portion of the cyst is delineated by marking the skin. (Either a wax pencil or a felt-tip marker is suitable for marking.)

may be detected in a person with thin musculature as the result of fluid gravitating along the long head of the biceps in the intertubercular synovial sheath (Fig. 7–1) and causing abnormal fullness in this area. Swelling or distention of the subacromial bursa may produce localized fullness under the deltoid muscle, which may be accentuated by partial passive abduction of the arm, since part of the bursa is compressed in this position (Fig. 7–4). Active abduction of the shoulder joint interferes with palpation of an enlarged subacromial bursa. Effusion of the suba-cromial bursa may be due to localized disease of the bursa or may repre-sent articular disease when the bursa communicates with the joint cavity. Occasionally, distention of the subcoracoid bursa may cause a small bulge just lateral to the coracoid process, and distention of the subcutaneous acromial bursa may cause swelling localized to the region just above the acromioclavicular joint.

Inspection and palpation are often combined in the examination of the shoulder.

PALPATION

Before the shoulder is examined by palpation, it is helpful to have the patient point out the area of maximal pain or tenderness by touching the involved shoulder with the hand of the uninvolved side. Since the patient cannot differentiate between referred pain to the shoulder and localized disease in the shoulder, the physician must utilize the examina-tion (as well as the history) to establish the source and nature of pain in the shoulder. Pain originating in the shoulder joint must be demonstra-ble locally and reproducibly by palpation or motion by the examiner when the patient can localize tenderness in order to differentiate it from pain referred to the shoulder because of extra-articular and potentially serious diseases (see p. 79). Sometimes the patient is unable to define a localized area of superficial tenderness and can only describe the area as "deep" in the general region of the shoulder. In such instances the pa-tient's vague localization is of relatively little diagnostic value, and the examiner must rely on evidence of localization obtained from the physi-cal examination.

If possible, the patient should be in either the sitting or the stand-ing position during examination. Initially, the examiner can best evaluate abnormalities of the shoulder by positioning himself in front of the pa-tient and palpating both shoulders for evidence of swelling, tenderness, local heat, muscle spasm, and atrophy. In this position and with this rou-tine he can compare the two shoulders easily. Then each shoulder can be examined from the side or posteriorly to obtain additional information.

A systematic examination of the shoulder includes palpation of the acromioclavicular joint (see p. 55), the rotator cuff, the region of the subacromial bursa, the intertubercular (bicipital) groove, and the anterior, lateral, and posterior aspects of the glenohumeral joint and the articular capsule. Palpation of the axilla for adenopathy and masses is also important.

Rotator Cuff

The posterior portion of the rotator cuff (tendons of infraspinatus and teres minor) is examined by having the patient adduct the arm across the chest and place the hand on the opposite shoulder. The examiner then stands in front of the patient and palpates the posterior surface of the humeral head by placing his thumb on the anterior aspect and his fingers on the posterior aspect of the patient's shoulder; the posterior portion of the rotator cuff is then beneath the examiner's fingers. The anterior portion of the cuff (subscapularis tendon) is examined by placing the patient's arm in backward extension (drawn backward about 20 degrees from the axillary line while the arm is still in adduction) and by palpating it anteriorly over the humeral head. If the examiner then stands behind the patient and places his fingers over the head of the humerus anteriorly while the patient internally rotates the arm by bringing his hand backward to a point between the scapulae, the superior portion of the rotator cuff (supraspinatus tendon) will be under the examiner's fingers and can be felt to move. During these maneuvers the examiner palpates the tendinous cuff for tenderness, swelling, firm nodular masses, or actual gaps (tears) in the cuff. Occasionally, he can palpate a soft, tender swelling that may represent the remaining proximal stub of a ruptured tendon attached to the humerus.

Degenerative lesions and abnormal calcium deposits in the rotator cuff frequently produce pain and tenderness over the upper portion of the humerus on the lateral aspect of the arm near the greater tubercle. In contrast, bicipital lesions cause maximal tenderness over the anterior portion of the humerus in the region of the intertubercular (bicipital) groove (see p. 69).

Articular Capsule, Synovial Membrane, and Glenohumeral Joint

The fibrous articular capsule of the shoulder is so closely associated with the tendons of the rotator cuff that both of these structures must be palpated simultaneously, since it is not possible to discriminate between them (as described in the previous section on palpation of the rotator cuff). If synovitis or effusion of the glenohumeral joint is detectable, a fluctuant distention is usually palpable, or warmth may be noticed over the anterior portion of the articular capsule and synovial membrane; however, the posterior portion of the capsule should also be palpated. Sometimes an effusion

of the shoulder joint may cause palpable swelling along the bicipital extension of the synovial membrane in the intertubercular (bicipital) groove
(Fig. 7–1). When the margins of the synovial membrane or articular capsule
are palpable, a moderate to considerable amount of synovitis or effusion is
present. Lesser effusions can sometimes be palpated by ballottement of
the anterior and lateral aspects of the shoulder alternately. Minimal degrees
of synovitis of the shoulder joint are not palpable.

Bursae Adjacent to the Shoulder

Inflammation or irritation of the subacromial (subdeltoid) bursa
may result in palpable swelling, tenderness, and warmth of the upper
portion of the arm in the region of the deltoid muscle and just distal to
the acromion process. Inflammation is usually associated with degenerative lesions or calcium deposits in the rotator cuff. Since a communication between the articular cavity and the subacromial bursa may occur,
effusion of the joint may sometimes be detected by swelling and distention
of the subacromial bursa. Pain related to the subacromial bursa is frequently
located near the insertion of the deltoid muscle, somewhat below the actual
site of the lesion.

Bicipital Groove

Inflammation of the synovial sheath or the tendon of the long
head of the biceps muscle (bicipital tenosynovitis) produces pain in the
region of the intertubercular (bicipital) groove. The pain may extend
along the biceps muscle into the arm. The condition is best detected by
palpation over the intertubercular (bicipital) groove, which extends along
the anterior aspect of the upper end of the humerus (Fig. 7–1). Palpation
is performed while the patient's arm and forearm are rotated externally
and with the examiner's fingers placed anteriorly over the groove to localize pain and to ascertain any tenderness, crepitus, or swelling in this
region. Sometimes tenderness in this area may be increased considerably
by rolling the bicipital tendon under the finger tips. If desired, the examiner may place his thumb posteriorly behind the arm to stabilize the examining fingers. The bicipital tendon and groove on the opposite side are
palpated for comparison.

If the patient's elbow is held at his side and flexed at a right angle
while the forearm is supinated against resistance supplied by the examiner's hand, pain will often be produced in the bicipital groove if tendinitis
or tenosynovitis is present (Yergason's sign). Another maneuver useful in
localizing involvement to the bicipital tendon is performed by passively
extending the elbow while the patient's hand and forearm are in the position of supination and the shoulder is passively moved posteriorly into a

hyperextended position. A positive response to this maneuver is indicated by the localization of pain in the bicipital groove. Flexion of the elbow, against resistance applied by the examiner, or active anterior flexion of the shoulder with the arm extended against resistance also may cause pain over the anterior portion of the arm and along the biceps tendon if an abnormality of the bicipital tendon is present.

MOVEMENT AND RANGE OF MOTION

Motion of the upper extremity on the trunk is normally a combination of movement of the shoulder girdle and the shoulder joint. The ball-and-socket shoulder joint is capable of a wide variety of movement. It permits flexion (forward movement of the arm), extension (dorsal flexion or backward movement of the arm), abduction (elevation of the arm from the side), adduction (lowering the arm to the side), rotation, and circumduction. The movements of the shoulder girdle as a whole on the chest wall include elevation (raising or shrugging the shoulder girdle above the normal resting position), depression (downward motion of the shoulder girdle below the normal resting position), protrusion (advancement of the shoulder girdle in front of the coronal plane), retraction (backward motion of the shoulder girdle behind the coronal plane), and circumduction.

Elevation of the arm from the side of the body (abduction) up over the head is accomplished by the combined movement of the shoulder joint and rotation of the scapula on the chest wall. This movement also is associated with motion of the sternoclavicular and acromioclavicular joints. Although there has been a tendency to separate active abduction of the arm into two distinct parts consisting of elevation of the arm to the horizontal position (using the glenohumeral joint) and raising of the arm from the horizontal position overhead (using scapulothoracic motion), such a distinction is artificial in normal active use of the shoulder, since both joints participate throughout abduction of the arm. As active normal elevation of the arm begins, only slight motion of the scapula occurs until the arm is in about 30 degrees of abduction. Thereafter, rotation of the scapula becomes more marked as the arm is raised over the head; after about 30 degrees of abduction, however, the glenohumeral joint contributes up to twice as much to abduction as scapular motion does. The relatively active normal movement of the shoulder joint and the scapulothoracic articulation may vary considerably in different individuals during abduction of the arm. When motion of the glenohumeral joint is limited by disease or muscle spasm, the individual may compensate by elevation of the entire shoulder girdle, using a hunching motion in an effort to abduct the arm more completely (Fig. 7–7).

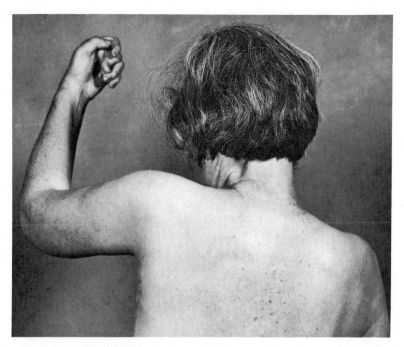

Figure 7–7. Limited abduction of left shoulder and severe flexion contractures of the fingers in a patient with shoulder-hand syndrome.

Four simple maneuvers may be used as an introductory or screening procedure for evaluation of the range of motion of the shoulder:

1. The patient is asked to extend both elbows fully (at the sides of the body) and then to move both the arms upward in wide vertical arcs (forward flexion or forward elevation) in an effort to touch the palmar surface of both hands together above the head (Fig. 7–8).

2. The patient is asked to touch both hands on the top of his head with the elbows flexed and the upper extremities moving in a horizontal arc posteriorly.

3. The patient is asked to raise each extended arm above his head in a wide sideways arc in the coronal plane of the body (abduction), finally attempting to touch the palmar surfaces of his hands together above his head with arms and forearms fully extended (Fig. 7–9). Some patients can accomplish this maneuver better when only one upper extremity is tested at a time or when the palms are turned up during abduction of the arm. When it is important to avoid the interference of set muscle antagonists, abduction can be tested better if the elbow is flexed before abduction is started.

4. The patient is asked to rotate his arm internally behind his back and place the back of his hand as high as possible between the scapulae (Fig. 7–10).

The relative contributions of scapular and humeral motions are

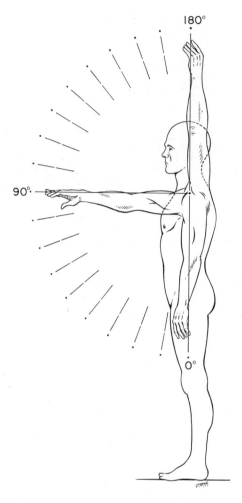

Figure 7–8. Forward flexion of extended arm with forearm also extended. This examination may be performed on each upper extremity separately or on both together. In the latter instance, the patient touches the palmar surface of both hands together over the head.

easily observed during these maneuvers by inspection or palpation or both of the patient from behind. Scapular motion also may be indicated by the degree of elevation of the shoulder. If this initial survey shows limitation of motion, the range of motion of the glenohumeral joint then needs to be examined in more detail.

Relatively little external rotation of the humerus is required when the arm is elevated over the head by forward flexion, whereas external rotation of about 180 degrees occurs when elevation of the arm is performed by abduction in a sideways arc over the head and then touching the palmar surfaces of the hands together. Thus, lesions affecting the rotating musculature of the humerus or the rotator cuff may cause pain, muscle spasm, or limitation of motion on abduction of the arm, while the range of forward flexion of the arm may remain relatively normal. Forward flexion of the arm is often a more reliable indication of the extent of shoulder motion than abduction is, since patients with muscle spasm and misuse of antagonist muscles may either restrict abduction of the arm or elevate the arm slowly, whereas they are able to accomplish the forward flexion with relative ease.

The motions that are of most value in the evaluation of the normal function of the glenohumeral joint are internal rotation, external rotation, and abduction. For accurate measurement of glenohumeral abduction, motion of the scapula should be prevented. This is best accomplished if the examiner grasps the inferior portion of the scapula and holds it firmly in place with one hand while he passively and slowly abducts the patient's arm with his other hand and forearm. The muscles of the abducted arm must be relaxed. This can be achieved by allowing

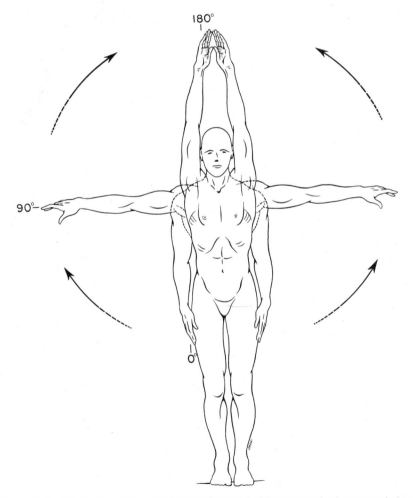

Figure 7–9. Abduction of both extended arms in a sideways arc in the coronal plane of the body, touching the palmar surface of the hands together above the head.

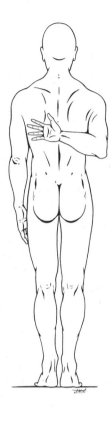

Figure 7-10. Position of right hand and arm placed behind the back in test of range of internal rotation of right shoulder. The patient should place his hand as high as possible between the scapulae, and the range of motion in the two shoulders is compared.

the patient's arm and forearm to rest on the arm and forearm of the examiner while the examiner's arm is slowly elevated. When the patient or examiner detects the appearance of muscle spasm, the examiner should temporarily stop the motion and ask the patient to press his elbow slightly downward onto the examiner's arm. This will relax the spasm at least temporarily and permit further attempts at passive abduction. If the scapula is adequately stabilized during this procedure, there should be no elevation of the shoulder or shoulder girdle. The scapula can be partially but satisfactorily stabilized by exerting downward .and restricting pressure on the acromion to prevent elevation of the shoulder girdle. The normal range of abduction of the glenohumeral joint under these circumstances is about 90 degrees or slightly more from the 0-degree (neutral) position with the arm resting at the side (Fig. 7-11).

Since the scapula normally moves during rotation of the shoulder and thus is a component of usual shoulder function, the entire shoulder girdle may be allowed to participate in the measurement of rotation. Rotation of the arm is best demonstrated when the examiner places himself at the side of the patient, who is either sitting or standing. Then, with the patient's arm abducted to 90 degrees, the patient's elbow flexed at a right angle, and the forearm horizontal (0 degrees; Fig. 7-12), the forearm is moved upward (external rotation of the shoulder) and down-

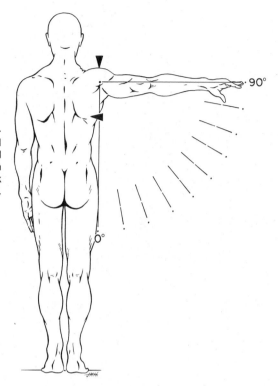

Figure 7–11. Range of abduction of the glenohumeral
joint with the scapula and
shoulder girdle stabilized in
the areas marked by the black
triangles. See text for details.

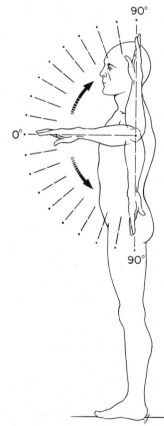

Figure 7–12. Range of internal and external rotation of the shoulder. With elbow bent at a right angle
and forearm held horizontally, the forearm is moved
upward for external rotation and downward for internal rotation. This examination also can be done
while the patient is supine.

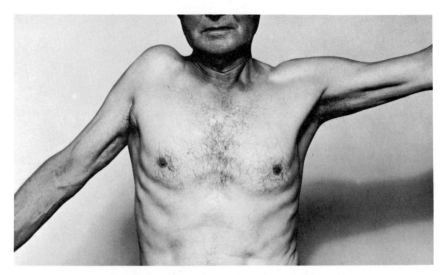

Figure 7–13. Partial tear of the rotator cuff of the right shoulder, with limitation of abduction of the arm and a characteristic hunched position of the involved shoulder as compared with abduction of the unaffected left shoulder.

ward (internal rotation of the shoulder). The normal range is about 90 degrees of internal rotation and 90 degrees of external rotation, as is shown in Figure 7–12.

Tears of the rotator cuff of the shoulder characteristically produce inability or limitation of active abduction of the arm from the side. Sometimes an individual with a partial tear of the rotator cuff can initiate abduction of the arm but is unable to raise it to a horizontal position. If the patient's arm is passively abducted to a horizontal position by the examiner, the patient then may have little or no difficulty in raising his arm over his head or lowering his arm to a horizontal position, but if the arm is lowered below a 90-degree angle, it may fall suddenly to the patient's side. Some individuals can hold the involved arm in a horizontal position when it is abducted by the examiner or by the patient's uninvolved arm, but the stability to maintain the arm in abduction against resistance applied in a downward direction by the examiner is distinctly impaired. Attempted abduction of the arm by a patient with a tear of the rotator cuff may produce a characteristic hunching motion of the shoulder, since the rotator cuff is unable to stabilize the humeral head adequately within the glenoid fossa of the scapula (Fig. 7–13).

Degenerative lesions of the rotator cuff often cause pain that starts when the arm is in about 70 degrees of abduction and disappears after the arm is raised above 100 degrees of abduction, since the acromion process tends to impinge on the rotator cuff and subacromial bursa between these degrees of motion in abduction (Fig. 7–4).

When secondary adhesive capsulitis (frozen shoulder) has developed, the cause of the original abnormality is often obscured. Initial physical examination of the shoulder alone may not permit differentiation of tears of the musculotendinous cuff, reflex dystrophy, rheumatoid arthritis, and other types of involvement of the shoulder that can result in a frozen shoulder.

MUSCLE TESTING

In most instances, the muscles of the shoulder joint can be tested sufficiently with the patient in the sitting position and the examiner sitting or standing at the side of the patient.

Flexion. The prime movers of flexion of the shoulder are the anterior portion of the deltoid muscle (axillary nerve, C5, 6) and the coracobrachialis muscle (musculocutaneous nerve, C5, 6). The accessory muscles to flexion are the middle fibers of the deltoid, the clavicular fibers of the pectoralis major, and the biceps brachii. To test flexion of the shoulder, the examiner immobilizes the patient's scapula as much as possible on the side being tested by grasping and holding the lower border with one hand. The patient then flexes (elevates) the arm anteriorly to 90 degrees with the forearm pronated and the elbow slightly flexed against graded resistance applied by the examiner's other hand just above the elbow, as illustrated in Figure 7–14. Rotation, adduction, or abduction of the arm should be prevented while flexion is being tested,

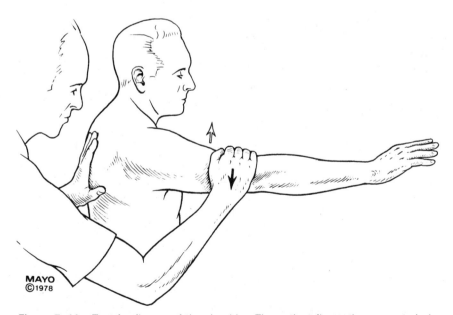

MAYO
©1978

Figure 7–14. Test for flexors of the shoulder. The patient flexes the arm anteriorly from his side while the examiner fixes the scapula with one hand and resists flexion with the other hand above the patient's elbow.

as these movements would permit the accessory muscles to substitute for the prime movers in the action.

Extension. The prime movers of shoulder extension are the latissimus dorsi (thoracodorsal nerve, C6–8), teres major (lowest subscapular nerve, C5, 6), and deltoid (axillary nerve, C5, 6) muscles. The teres minor and long head of the triceps muscles are accessory to this motion. Extension of the shoulder is tested with the patient's elbow straightened and the forearm fully pronated (palm posterior) to prevent lateral rotation and adduction. The examiner fixes the scapula as described for testing flexion, and the patient extends the arm posteriorly through the range of extension against graded resistance provided by the examiner's other hand just above the patient's elbow.

Abduction. The prime movers of abduction are the middle fibers of the deltoid (axillary nerve, C5, 6) and the supraspinatus (suprascapular nerve, C5) muscles. The accessory muscles in abduction are the anterior and posterior fibers of the deltoid and serratus anterior muscles. The latter functions by direct action on the scapula. Abduction of the shoulder is tested with the patient's arm at his side, the forearm midway between pronation and supination (palm medial), and the elbow flexed a few degrees. The examiner stabilizes the scapula as described for flexion. The patient abducts the arm to 90 degrees against graded resistance applied by the examiner's other hand proximal to the patient's elbow.

Horizontal Abduction. The prime mover of horizontal abduction is the posterior portion of the deltoid muscle (axillary nerve, C5, 6). The infraspinatus and teres minor are the accessory muscles to this motion. Horizontal abduction occurs mainly at the glenohumeral joint and is tested with the patient's shoulder abducted to 90 degrees. The examiner stabilizes the scapula as previously described, and the patient is instructed to move his arm horizontally and posteriorly against graded resistance applied by the examiner's other hand proximal to the patient's elbow (Fig. 7–15).

Horizontal Adduction. The prime mover of horizontal adduction of the shoulder is the pectoralis major muscle (medial and lateral pectoral nerves, C5–8, T1); the anterior fibers of the deltoid muscle are accessory to this motion. Horizontal adduction also occurs mainly at the glenohumeral joint and is assessed with the patient's arm abducted to 90 degrees. The patient adducts the arm anteriorly through the horizontal plane of motion against graded resistance applied by the examiner's other hand placed over the front of the arm just proximal to the patient's elbow.

Lateral Rotation. The prime movers of lateral rotation are the infraspinatus (suprascapular nerve, C5, 6) and teres minor (axillary nerve, C5) muscles; the posterior fibers of the deltoid muscle are accessory to this motion. The lateral rotation of the shoulder is assessed with the patient's arm abducted to 90 degrees (or at the patient's side if abduction is not possible), with the elbow flexed to 90 degrees, and the hand and

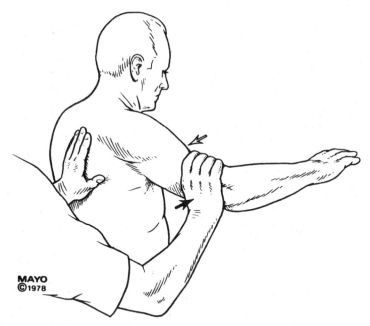

Figure 7–15. Test for horizontal abductors of the shoulder. With the shoulder abducted to 90 degrees, the patient abducts the arm posteriorly while the examiner stabilizes the scapula with one hand and resists horizontal abduction with the other hand proximal to the elbow.

fingers pointing forward. The examiner supports the patient's elbow by holding it with one hand while the patient rotates the arm upward (or outward if shoulder abduction is not possible) against graded resistance applied by the examiner's other hand on the patient's forearm proximal to the wrist.

Medial Rotation. The prime movers of medial rotation of the shoulder are the subscapularis (upper and lower subscapular nerves, C5, 6), pectoralis major (medial and lateral pectoral nerves, C5–8, T1), and teres major (lowest subscapular nerve, C5, 6) muscles; the anterior fibers of the deltoid muscle are accessory to this motion. Medial rotation of the shoulder is tested with the arm abducted to 90 degrees (or at the patient's side if abduction is not possible), the elbow flexed to 90 degrees, and the hand pointing forward. The examiner supports the patient's elbow with one hand as described previously while the patient rotates the arm downward (or inward if shoulder abduction is not possible) against graded resistance applied by the examiner's other hand on the patient's forearm proximal to the wrist.

REFERRED PAIN

Many disease processes in areas other than the shoulder may cause pain in the shoulder region and can be confused with involvement of the shoulder or adjacent structures. Cardiac disease, involvement of the pleura, and hiatal hernia all may produce pain that is referred to the shoulder. Subphrenic inflammation may irritate the inferior portion of the diaphragm and produce referred pain and tenderness in the region of the neck and shoulder. Diseases of the cervical portion of the spinal column, nerve roots, or peripheral nerves in the upper extremity are frequent extraneous sources of shoulder pain and disability. Sometimes they may cause difficulty in the recognition and interpretation of symptoms in the region of the shoulder. When pain in the shoulder is not related to use of the joint and the examination indicates a completely normal shoulder, referred pain should be considered as a possible cause of the symptoms.

SUGGESTED READING FOR ADDITIONAL INFORMATION

1. Moseley HF: Shoulder Lesions. Third edition. Baltimore, Williams & Wilkins Company, 1969, 318 pp.
2. Bateman JE: The Shoulder and Neck. Second edition. Philadelphia, WB Saunders Company, 1978, 850 pp.
3. De Palma AF: Surgery of the Shoulder. Second edition, Philadelphia, JB Lippincott Company, 1973, 551 pp.
4. Bland JH, Merrit JA, Boushey DR: The painful shoulder. Semin Arthritis Rheum 7:21–47, 1977.
5. Lucas DB: Biomechanics of the shoulder joint. Arch Surg 107:425–432, 1973.

chapter **8**

The Elbow

ESSENTIAL ANATOMY

The elbow is a hinge joint formed by the humero-ulnar, radiohumeral, and proximal radio-ulnar articulations. Thus, the elbow actually is composed of three bony articulations, the principal one of which is the humero-ulnar. All of these bony junctions are enclosed by the articular capsule in a common synovial articular cavity. Thus, the synovial membrane of the elbow is relatively extensive. Proximally, it is attached at the margin of the articular surface of the humerus and is reflected upward, lining the coronoid and radial fossae anteriorly and the olecranon fossa posteriorly. It is reflected downward from this area to its attachment at the margin of the articular surfaces of the ulna and radius. There are three masses of fat between the synovial membrane and the overlying capsule. The largest lies over the olecranon fossa; the others lie over the coronoid fossa and the radial fossa. Since the synovial membrane is usually palpable only posteriorly, only the posterior aspect of the elbow is illustrated in Figure 8–1. The articular capsule is thickened laterally and medially to form the radial collateral and ulnar collateral ligaments. The para-olecranon grooves are the spaces between the olecranon process of the ulna and the medial and lateral epicondyles of the humerus.

One large bursa (olecranon) and several small bursae lie about the elbow. The latter are not uniformly present, and neither the olecranon

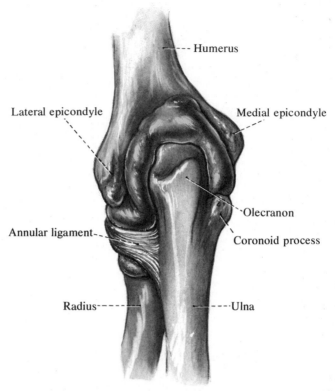

Figure 8–1. Posterior aspect of elbow joint showing radius and ulna in extension and distribution of synovial membrane in distention.

nor the other bursae communicate with the joint cavity under normal conditions.

INSPECTION

The elbows are best inspected while the patient is either sitting or standing. When this is not possible, the elbow of a patient in a supine position is examined by raising the shoulder forward 10 to 20 degrees and placing the arm across the patient's chest in as comfortable a position as possible. Medial and lateral deviations of the forearm on the arm are called "cubitus varus" and "cubitus valgus," respectively. When subluxation of the elbow occurs, the forearm is usually dislocated posteriorly in relation to the humerus (Fig. 8–2). Anterior subluxation of the forearm would include fracture of the olecranon process. Swelling and redness of the olecranon bursa are easily observed because of the close proximity of this bursa to the skin (Fig. 8–3). Common sites for subcutaneous nodules are in the olecranon bursa and along the extensor or most exposed surface of the ulna distal to the olecranon process (Fig. 8–4). When there is

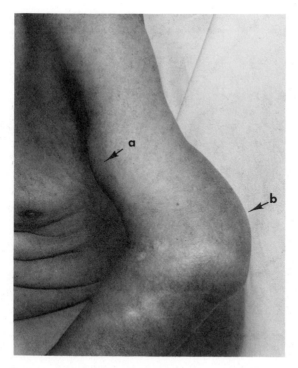

Figure 8–2. Charcot's arthropathy of left elbow of a patient with tabes dorsalis showing severe subluxation and deformity. The humerus protrudes anteriorly *(a)* and the ulna posteriorly *(b)* above the level of the elbow.

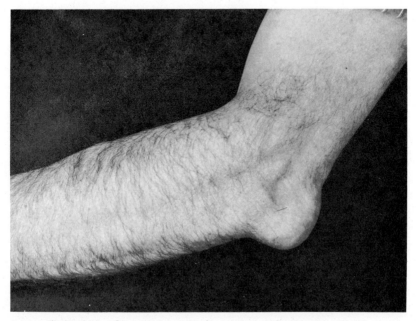

Figure 8–3. Olecranon bursitis in a patient with tophaceous gout.

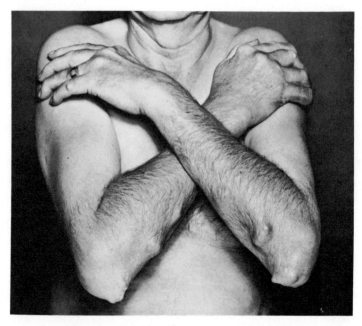

Figure 8–4. Subcutaneous nodules on the extensor surface of both forearms and hands in a patient with rheumatoid arthritis.

effusion or synovial thickening in the joint, the condition is usually first apparent as a bulge or fullness in the para-olecranon grooves on each side of the olecranon process (Fig. 8–5).

PALPATION

Synovial Membrane

The elbow joint may be palpated with the patient in either the supine or sitting position, but the elbow should be as relaxed as possible. Irrespective of the position of the patient, the examiner will use his left hand to give firm support to the left forearm of the patient while his right thumb and fingers palpate the left elbow. The right elbow is examined in the same fashion except that the examiner palpates with his left thumb and fingers and uses his right hand to support the forearm. As shown in Figure 8–6, the thumb is placed over the lateral para-olecranon groove, and the forefinger or middle finger or both are placed over the medial para-olecranon groove. These spaces are best palpated with the patient's elbow flexed about 70 degrees from the position of complete extension and with the muscles relaxed. Synovial thickening or joint effusion or both are more often palpable in the medial than in the lateral para-olecranon groove but should be discernible on palpation in both because of the anatomic distribution of the synovial membrane in this joint (Fig. 8–1). The pressure of the examining fingers and thumb should be varied while these digits palpate the para-olecranon grooves. A soft, boggy, or fluctuant fullness in both grooves indicates synovial thickening or effusion or both and can be differentiated from the more solid consistency of the adjacent fat pads and other soft tissues. Local heat or redness, if present, often extends beyond the confines of the synovial membrane. Slowly extending the patient's arm while the examiner keeps his thumb and fingers in the para-olecranon grooves often helps the examiner to identify synovitis. The synovial membrane may bulge under the palpating thumb or fingers as the forearm is extended. This maneuver also helps the examiner distinguish tendons, muscles, fat pads, and ligaments from the synovial membrane in this area. Occasionally, the differentiation of synovial thickening from effusion may be suggested by palpation of the synovial membrane over the posterior bony margins of the radiohumeral joint.

The elbow is a common site of synovitis, but this involvement is often overlooked. In the detection of synovitis by physical examination it is particularly helpful to compare the physical findings of a suspected abnormal joint with those of a normal joint. Synovitis of the elbow also is commonly associated with limitation of extension of the joint.

Other Tissues

The *olecranon bursa* can be palpated easily for fluid, swelling, tenderness, local heat, consistency, loose bodies, and nodules. Nodules,

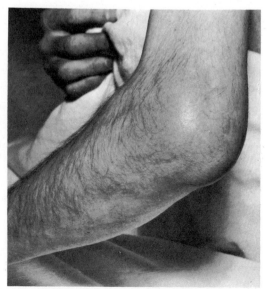

Figure 8–5. Acute gouty arthritis of the elbow showing swelling of the synovial membrane and perisynovial tissues on the posterior aspect of the joint.

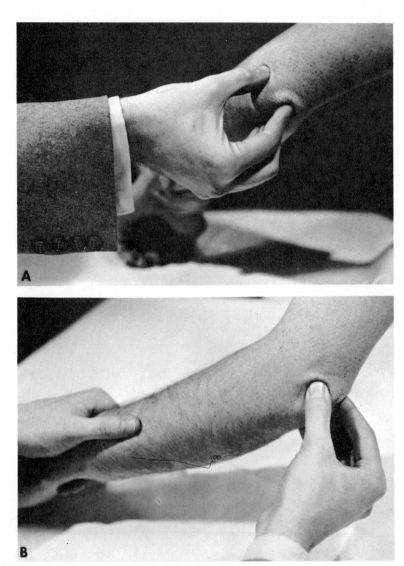

Figure 8–6. Palpation for synovial thickening or effusion of left elbow. *A.* Posterior view. *B.* Side view. The examiner's left hand is supporting the forearm with the elbow flexed about 70 degrees from the position of complete extension. The examiner's right thumb and fingers are used to palpate between the lateral and medial edges of the olecranon process and the humeral epicondyles. See text for details.

loose bodies, and tenderness are most apparent with the elbow fully flexed, whereas the bursa and adjacent tissues may be palpated best between the examiner's thumb and second finger with the patient's elbow extended. If the olecranon bursa is enlarged, the bursa may or may not be fixed to the underlying olecranon process.

Subcutaneous nodules may be large enough to be seen, but some that are not can be palpated when the examiner runs his finger along the extensor surface of the ulna. Nodules are detected as raised, firm, non-tender nodes on the extensor surface of the ulna in or distal to the ole-cranon bursa. The overlying skin and subcutaneous tissues can be moved freely over a subcutaneous nodule, but the mobility of the nodule itself depends on its location. When a nodule is in the olecranon bursa, it is relatively more movable than when it is in the subcutaneous tissues or affixed to the periosteum. Slight bony irregularities of the ulnar surface may be present in this area and are not abnormal.

The *medial and lateral epicondyles* of the humerus, the head of the radius, and the tendinous attachments of muscles to these structures are common sites of inflammation, pain, or localized tenderness ("tennis elbow" or "epicondylitis"). The ulnar nerve and groove also can be pal-pated for indications of thickening, irregularity, and tenderness.

Swelling of the articular capsule occasionally may be detected by deep palpation of the antecubital space, but swelling in such instances is usually evident and more easily detected by the posterior examination of the elbow as described.

MOVEMENT AND RANGE OF MOTION

The position of complete extension of the elbow is designated here as 0 degrees. A few individuals normally lack 5 to 10 degrees of full extension, and others may have 5 to 10 degrees of hyperextension. When the joint is flexed, the angle between the arm and forearm nor-mally is 160 to 150 degrees of flexion from the extended position (Fig. 8–7). The movements of flexion and extension occur in the humero-ulnar and radiohumeral joints. Pronation and supination of the hand and

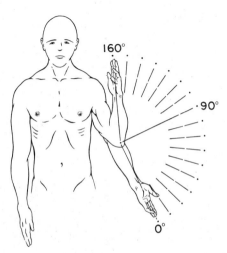

Figure 8–7. Range of normal flexion (0 to 150 or 160 degrees) and extension (150 or 160 to 0 degrees) of the elbow.

forearm involve motion of both radio-ulnar joints (at the elbow and the wrist) and the radiohumeral joint. Normally, these joints allow approximately 180 degrees of movement that can be divided into about 90 degrees of pronation and about 90 degrees of supination from a position midway between the two extremes (Fig. 8–8).

MUSCLE TESTING

Flexion. The prime movers in flexion of the elbow are the biceps brachii (musculocutaneous nerve, C5, 6), brachialis (musculocutaneous nerve, C5, 6), and brachioradialis (radial nerve, C5, 6) muscles. The flexor muscles of the forearm arising from the medial epicondyle of the humerus are the accessory muscles. For testing flexion of the elbow, the patient sits with the arm at his side and the forearm supinated. The examiner stabilizes the patient's arm by grasping it with one hand, as shown in Figure 8–9. The patient is then instructed to flex the elbow through its range of motion against graded resistance applied by the examiner's other hand just proximal to the patient's wrist.

Extension. The prime mover in extension of the elbow is the triceps brachii muscle (radial nerve, C7, 8); the anconeus muscle is an accessory. To test extension of the elbow, the examiner fixes the patient's arm as described for flexion, and the patient is instructed to move his elbow through the range of extension against graded resistance provided by the examiner's other hand just proximal to the patient's wrist.

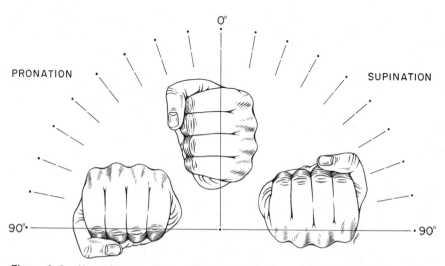

Figure 8–8. Normal range of pronation and supination of the hand and forearm. In this diagram the fingers are flexed to form a fist, but the examination can be made with the patient's fingers extended or semiflexed.

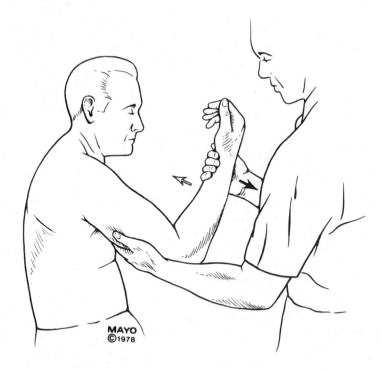

Figure 8–9. Test for flexors of the elbow. The patient flexes the elbow while the examiner stabilizes the arm with one hand without causing pain and resists flexion with the other hand proximal to the wrist.

SUGGESTED READING FOR ADDITIONAL INFORMATION

1. Smith FM: Surgery of the Elbow. Second edition. Philadelphia, WB Saunders Company, 1972, 340 pp.
2. Porter BB, Richardson C, Vainio K: Rheumatoid arthritis of the elbow: The results of synovectomy. J Bone Joint Surg [Br] 56B:427–437, 1974.
3. Murray-Leslie CF, Wright V: Carpal tunnel syndrome, humeral epicondylitis, and the cervical spine: A study of clinical and dimensional relations. Br Med J 1:1439–1442, 1976.

chapter **9**

The Wrist and Carpal Joints

ESSENTIAL ANATOMY

Joints and Synovial Membranes

Wrist or Radiocarpal Articulation. The wrist joint is formed proximally by the distal end of the radius and the articular disk and distally by a row of carpal bones, the scaphoid (formerly called the "navicular"), the lunate, and the triangular (alternatively called "triquetrum" or "triquetral"; Fig. 9–1). The articular disk joins the radius to the ulna and separates the distal end of the ulna from the wrist joint proper. The wrist joint is surrounded by a capsule and supported by ligaments. The synovial membrane lines the inner surface of the articular capsule. The capsule and underlying synovial membrane are loose, especially over the dorsum of the wrist where the distal ends of the radius and ulna lie near the surface under the skin.

Distal Radio-ulnar Joint. This joint is adjacent to the radiocarpal joint (wrist joint) but usually is not a part of it, since the articular disk divides these joints into two separate cavities (Fig. 9–1). The synovial membrane loosely lines the deep surface of the articular capsule and internal ligaments and bulges upward between the radius and ulna beyond the level of the articular surfaces.

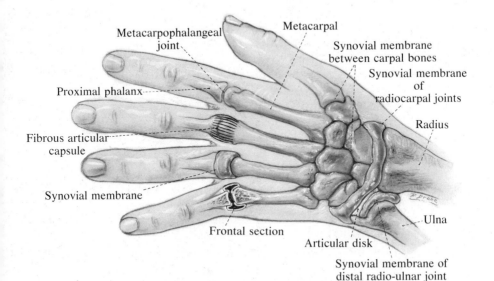

Figure 9–1. Relationship of the synovial membranes of the wrist, carpal, and metacarpophalangeal joints to adjacent bony and surface landmarks. The carpal bones in the distal row, listed sequentially from the radial to the ulnar sides, are trapezium, trapezoid, capitate, and hamate. In the proximal row in the same sequence the bones are scaphoid, lunate, and triangular (or triquetrum or triquetral). The pisiform, which is not seen on the dorsal aspect, articulates with the triangular on the palmar aspect of the wrist.

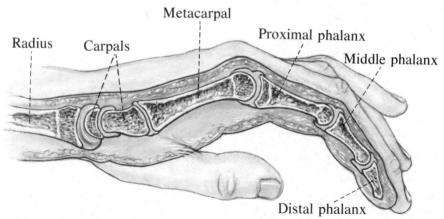

Figure 9–2. Sagittal section through wrist and hand showing location of synovial membranes. Note that the synovial membrane extends farther proximally than distally at the metacarpophalangeal and interphalangeal joints.

Midcarpal Joint. The midcarpal joint is formed by the junction of the proximal and distal rows of carpal bones. It permits some flexion and extension and a slight amount of rotation. The midcarpal and carpometacarpal articular cavities often communicate and are lined with a synovial membrane, which covers the deep surfaces of the intercarpal ligaments and the surrounding capsule (Figs. 9–1 and 9–2).

Tendons and Synovial Sheaths of the Wrist and Hand; the Median Nerve

The synovial tendon sheaths of the wrist and hand will be discussed together.

Flexor Tendons. The long flexor tendons of the muscles of the forearm are enclosed in a common flexor tendon sheath (sometimes called the "ulnar bursa"), which begins about 2.5 cm proximal to the wrist crease and extends to the midpalm. The tendon sheath of the flexor pollicis longus may be completely separate or may join the sheath of the common flexor tendon (Fig. 9–3). Part of the common flexor tendon sheath lies in a fibro-osseous canal (carpal tunnel) that is bounded anteriorly (palmar aspect) by the flexor retinaculum (transverse carpal ligament) and posteriorly (dorsal aspect) by the carpal bones and ligaments on the floor of the canal.

The flexor retinaculum is crossed anteriorly by the palmaris longus tendon and anteromedially by the ulnar nerve, ulnar artery, and ulnar vein. The latter three structures may have additional connective tissue covering them anteriorly (the volar carpal ligament or superficial part of the transverse carpal ligament), but this additional connective tissue is not involved in the production of the carpal tunnel syndrome.

Median Nerve. The median nerve also runs through the carpal tunnel. It lies between the anterior surface of the common flexor tendon sheath and the flexor retinaculum and may be compressed by the firm, unyielding flexor retinaculum if swelling or edema occurs in this region (Fig. 9–3).

The tendon sheath of the fifth finger is usually continuous with the common flexor tendon sheath, whereas the common flexor tendon sheath covering the tendons of the second (index), third (middle), and fourth (ring) fingers ends at midpalm. The flexor tendons then continue distally without a tendon sheath until covered individually by their respective digital synovial sheaths (Fig. 9–3).

Palmar Aponeurosis. The palmar aponeurosis (fascia) begins at the level of the retinaculum as the apex of a triangle that fans out into the central portion of the palm. The apex of the aponeurosis is a direct continuation of the tendon of the palmaris longus. The central portion has thickened bands that lie over the flexor tendons and extend into the digits. The four bands to the second (index), third (middle), fourth (ring),

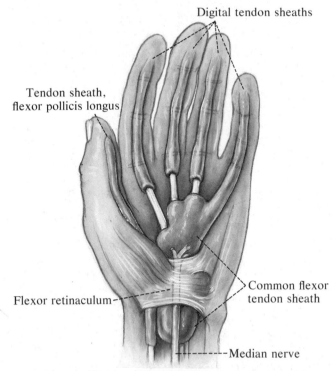

Figure 9–3. Anterior (palmar) aspect of the wrist and digits showing the distribution of the synovial sheaths of the flexor tendons. The median nerve lies between the anterior surface of the common flexor tendon sheath and the flexor retinaculum, where it is subject to compression by the firm, unyielding retinaculum if swelling occurs in this region.

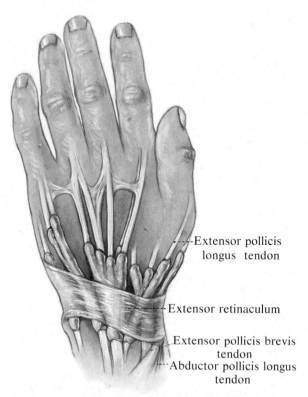

-----Extensor pollicis
          longus tendon

-----Extensor retinaculum

_Extensor pollicis brevis
          tendon
---Abductor pollicis longus
          tendon

Figure 9–4. Posterior (dorsal) aspect of the wrist showing the distribution of the synovial sheaths of the extensor tendons. The extensor pollicis brevis and the abductor pollicis longus, the principal tendons involved in stenosing tenosynovitis at the radial styloid process, are identified.

and fifth (little) fingers are thicker and more constant than the one to the thumb.

  Extensor Tendons. The extensor tendons of the forearm pass through six fibro-osseous tunnels on the dorsum of the wrist. These tunnels are bound superficially by the extensor retinaculum (dorsal carpal ligament) and on the deep surface by the carpal bones and ligaments. Each tunnel is lined with a synovial sheath that extends about 2.5 cm proximally and distally from the extensor retinaculum (Fig. 9–4). The long abductor and short extensor tendons of the thumb pass through the most radial of the six fibro-osseous tunnels. These tendons pass the prominence of the radial styloid process and thus are subject to particular friction and trauma at this site. A triangular depression over the dorsolateral aspect of the wrist that is visible when the thumb is extended and abducted is known as the anatomic "snuffbox." In this anatomic position the tendons of the abductor pollicis longus and extensor pollicis brevis muscles form the lateral boundary, and the tendon of the extensor pollicis longus muscle forms the medial boundary. The anatomic "snuffbox" is limited proximally by the radial styloid process and distally by the base of the metacarpal bone of the thumb. The long extensor tendon of the thumb is particularly vulnerable to wear and fraying because it functions repeatedly over bony prominences. This tendon passes through a bony groove on the medial aspect of the dorsal tubercle of the scaphoid, where angulation caused by dorsiflexion or radial deviation may pull the tendon around a rough edge and also predispose it to rupture.

INSPECTION

Swelling of the Wrist

Swelling of the wrist may be localized or diffuse (Figs. 9–5 and 9–6). Localized synovial swellings on the dorsum of the wrist may resemble cysts and result from synovial outpouchings of tendon sheaths or from outpouchings of the synovial membrane lining the wrist joint. In the latter instance the synovial swelling protrudes from under the extensor tendons. When articular synovial swelling is seen on the volar aspect of the wrist, it lies adjacent to the flexor tendons. Similar cystic synovial swelling may arise from the tendon sheaths in the hand and may be found anywhere in the hand, but it will be within the confines of the tendon sheath or sheaths involved.

Ganglion. The term "ganglion" (plural, ganglia or ganglions) is used commonly to describe a cystic enlargement that characteristically occurs on the dorsal surface of the wrist between the tendons of the common extensors of the digits and the radial extensors at the base of

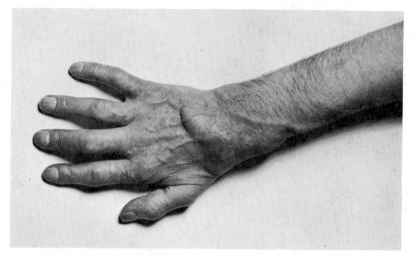

Figure 9–5. Cystic synovial outpouching on the dorsum of the wrist associated with tenosynovitis in a patient with rheumatoid arthritis.

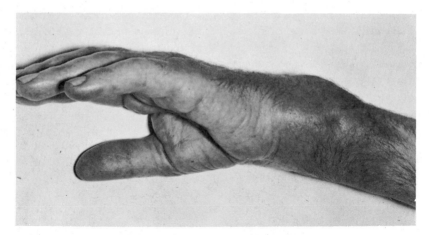

Figure 9–6. Diffuse swelling, edema, and induration accompanying staphylococcal arthritis of the wrist.

the second metacarpal bone (Fig. 9–7). Other common sites for ganglia are the anatomic "snuffbox" at the base of the thumb on the dorsal aspect of the hand and on the radial side of the volar aspect of the wrist. Ganglia also may arise from the tendon sheaths of the flexor tendons over the proximal phalanges of the fingers, usually just beyond the distal palmar crease.

Ganglia arise from the joint capsule and may be considered benign tenosynovial tumors (Fig. 9–7). They do not communicate with the joint

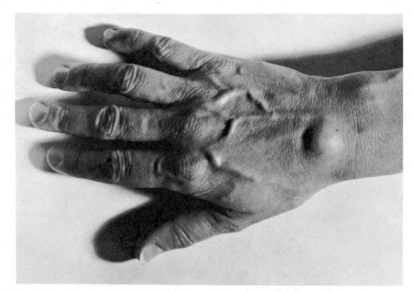

Figure 9–7. Ganglion or small cystic swelling on dorsum of right hand just distal to the wrist joint.

but do have a synovial lining membrane resembling that of diarthrodial joints, tendon sheaths, or bursae. Ganglia contain a thick mucoid or semi-solid material and may vary in size from those that are only barely visible on inspection to those that are several centimeters in diameter. The multiplanar motion associated with the scaphoid bone during movement of the wrist may be a predisposing factor to the formation of ganglia adjacent to the scaphoid-lunate articulation, as occurs frequently. Ganglia usually cause relatively few, if any, symptoms other than localized swelling and mild discomfort with motion, but they can become tender and painful when distended.

Deformity of the Wrist and Function of the Hand

Proper positioning of the wrist is essential for adequate function of the hand. When the wrist is flexed (palmar), much of the power of flexion in the fingers is lost. If the wrist is ankylosed or partially fixed in flexion, the hand loses some of its usefulness, because in this position the extensor tendons of the digits tend to extend the metacarpophalangeal joints and the thumb is extended and abducted, flattening this portion of the hand and making it difficult or impossible for the thumb to oppose the fingers (Fig. 9–8). At the same time, the interphalangeal joints become extended unless flexion contractures of the fingers have occurred. This is in contrast to the functional position of the hand when the wrist

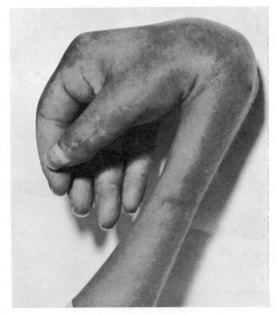

Figure 9–8. Ankylosis of the wrist in extreme flexion, resulting in a practically useless hand of a patient with severe rheumatoid arthritis.

is partially extended (dorsiflexion); in this instance, the fingers and meta-carpophalangeal joints can be flexed and the thumb positioned for opposing the fingers, producing useful hand function.

Other Abnormalities of the Wrist and Hand

In the usual deformity associated with thickening and contracture of the palmar aponeurosis (Dupuytren's contracture), the involved fingers are drawn into flexion contractures, first at the metacarpophalangeal joint, followed by flexion of the proximal interphalangeal joint. The fourth digit or ring finger is involved earliest, then the fifth and third digits in that order. The second and first digits are rarely affected. The skin may be irregularly bound down to the involved areas of the aponeurosis (Fig. 9–9).

Atrophy of thenar muscles suggests interference with the motor function of the median nerve at the wrist (carpal tunnel syndrome; Fig. 9–10). Abnormal dorsolateral prominence of the ulna indicates subluxation of the distal end of the ulna (Fig. 9–11). Subluxation of the ulna causes abnormal pressure on the extensor digitorum communis tendons, especially those of the fourth and fifth digits, and may result in rupture of these tendons (Fig. 9–12). Helpful information can be obtained by

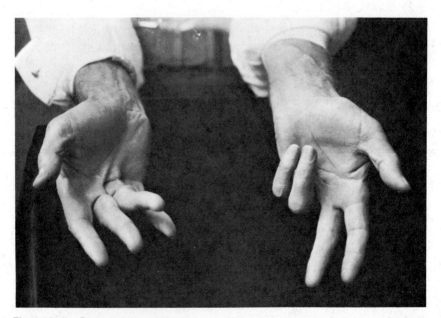

Figure 9–9. Dupuytren's contractures in both hands showing flexion contractures of the fourth and fifth digits of the left hand and less severe contractures in the third, fourth, and fifth digits of the right hand. Note the puckering of palmar skin and the presence of bands extending from the concavity of the palm to the proximal interphalangeal joints of the third and fourth digits of the right hand.

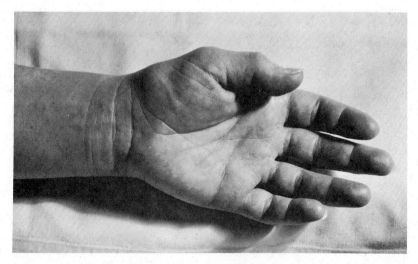

Figure 9–10. Atrophy of thenar muscles resulting from compression of the median nerve in the carpal tunnel (carpal tunnel syndrome).

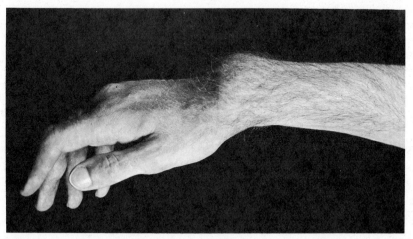

Figure 9–11. Subluxation of wrist with prominence of the dorsally protruding ulna resulting from severe rheumatoid arthritis. Moderate synovitis of wrist and muscular atrophy are also present.

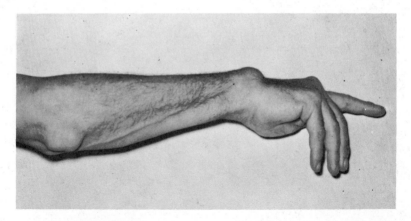

Figure 9–12. Dorsal dislocation of the ulna with resultant rupture of extensor tendons of third (middle), fourth (ring), and fifth (little) fingers of the right hand of a patient with rheumatoid arthritis.

recognizing abnormal conditions of the skin (for example, pale, clammy, sweaty, red, atrophic, or hidebound, abnormally tight skin) and the presence of nodules, scars of previous operation or trauma, cutaneous lesions, and atrophy of muscles proximal or distal to the wrist.

PALPATION

Wrist

Synovitis in the wrist is indicated by swelling or soft-tissue fullness, with or without tenderness and localized warmth, and is detected most reliably by palpation over the dorsum of the wrist. Because of overlying structures, accurate dorsal and volar localization of the margins of the synovial reflection in the wrist may be difficult. True articular swelling (synovitis) of the wrist is often most palpable just distal to the head (prominence) of the ulna on the dorsolateral aspect of the wrist when the palm is turned down. The synovial reflection is more extensive in this region than in other regions of the wrist (Fig. 9–1).

Palpation of the wrist may be accomplished by using either of two techniques:

1. The examiner faces the patient and supports the patient's hand with his fingers while palpating the wrist firmly (using two hands) by placing both thumbs on the dorsum of the wrist and both second (index) and third (middle) fingers on the volar aspect of the wrist (Fig. 9–13). The patient's wrist should be relaxed and in a straight position (0 degrees) with the palm turned down. The palpating thumbs are moved above and the palpating fingers below and from side to side over the depressed areas that lie over the region of the joint space just distal to

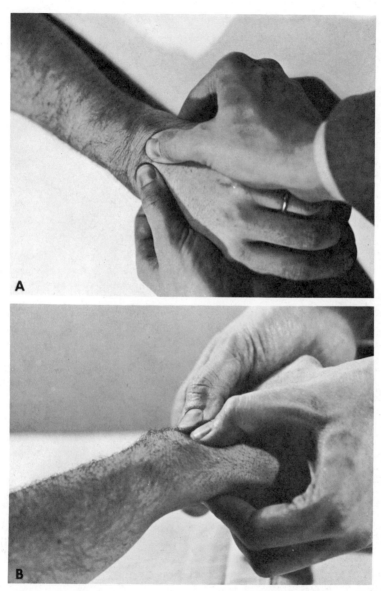

Figure 9–13. Palpation of the left wrist by using both hands. *A.* Top view. *B.* Side view. The wrist is being palpated firmly (note blanched nails of examiner's thumbs) by both thumbs and second (index) fingers. The other fingers serve to support and position the patient's hand as partially shown in *B.* See text for details.

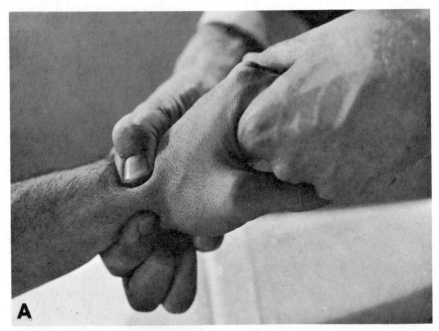

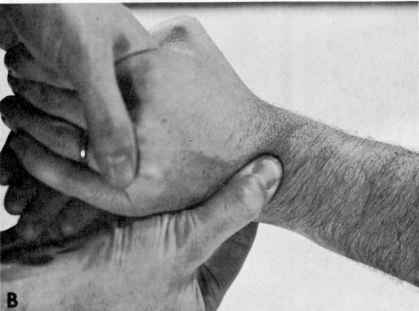

Figure 9–14. Palpation of the left wrist using one hand. The examiner's left hand is supporting the patient's hand and wrist in slight dorsiflexion while the examiner's right thumb and second (index) finger are used in pinching motions to examine the joint. *A.* Palpation of radial aspect of the joint. *B.* Palpation of midportion. *C.* Palpation of ulnar aspect of the wrist. The examiner palpates above and below the depressed area of the joint space while moving the examining thumb and fingers across the wrist from one side to the other. The blanched nail of the palpating thumb indicates that firm but gentle pressure is applied.

Illustration continued on opposite page.

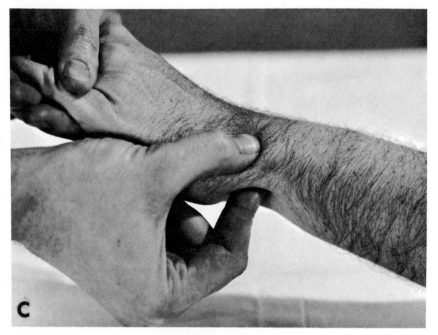

Figure 9–14. *Continued.*

the bony prominences of the radius and ulna. Gentle but firm pressure should be applied by the examining thumbs and fingers in order to detect adequately the bony and soft-tissue structures.

2. In an alternative method of examining the wrist, the physician supports the patient's hand with one hand while the patient's wrist remains relaxed and in a straight position (0 degrees) or slightly dorsiflexed, with the palm turned down. With his other hand the examining physician then palpates the patient's wrist firmly between his thumb and fingers by placing his thumb on the dorsum of the wrist and his second (index) and third (middle) fingers on the volar aspect of the wrist (Fig. 9–14). The examiner palpates proximal and distal to the depressed areas of the joint space while moving the examining fingers and thumb across the wrist from one side to the other.

The soft-tissue swelling of synovitis in the wrist can be evaluated further by examining the radial aspect of the wrist to detect a palpable bulge when the ulnar side of the wrist joint is compressed.

Sometimes compression of a dorsally located cystic swelling will demonstrate its communication with the wrist joint by causing distention of the articular capsule as the fluid in the cystic swelling is pushed back temporarily into the wrist joint cavity. If the cyst has resulted from an outpouching of a tendon sheath that does not communicate with the wrist joint, pressure over the cyst will cause distention only over the anatomic distribution of the involved tendon sheath. The close anatomic relationship between the tendon sheaths and the wrist joint often makes it difficult to differentiate localized tenosynovitis from articular synovitis at the level of the wrist. Swelling and tenderness localized to the region of the radial styloid process may result from stenosing tenosynovitis (de Quervain's tenosynovitis) in this area. Additional information also can be obtained by palpating the wrist for nodules on bones or tendons and for changes in skin temperature.

Hypertrophic Osteoarthropathy.   Hypertrophic osteoarthropathy may produce periostitis and periosteal proliferation near the ends of long bones. These often affect either unilaterally or bilaterally the distal part of the radius or ulna or both. Hypertrophic osteoarthropathy may be associated with advanced or severe clubbing or may occur without any definite clubbing of the nails (see pp. 120 and 133). The patient may or may not be aware of discomfort or soft-tissue swelling in the affected area or areas. Such swelling, if present, occurs proximal to the wrist joint, is usually slight or mild, and is not well localized to the distal part of the forearm. It lacks the typical consistency of either synovial swelling or pitting edema. When pain is present (whether felt only during palpation or continuously), it is located over the affected long bones and is proximal to the wrist joint itself. The joint usually is free of discomfort and motion is not limited. On occasion, however, extreme or well-advanced hypertrophic osteoarthropathy may affect the joint. In the absence of definitive physical signs, only roentgenographic examination of the long bones of the forearm (or elsewhere) will reveal hypertrophic osteoarthropathy.

Palm of Hand and Carpal Joints

After examining the wrist, the examiner may move his fingers distally to palpate the palm and carpal joints. With the examining fingers in the patient's palm and the examining thumbs located on the dorsal aspect of the patient's hand, the physician uses pinching motions in palpating the carpal bones and joints for the presence and localization of swelling, tenderness, and crepitation. Swelling and tenderness in the joints of the carpal bones are often caused by either a mechanical injury or a specific infectious process if they occur without involvement of other joints of the hand or wrist. The localization of involved carpal joints is often difficult by physical examination, and the examiner may need to rely on x-ray changes for precise localization in this area.

Tenosynovitis; Trigger Finger.   When the patient's palm is lightly palpated by the examiner while the patient's fingers are slowly and actively flexed and extended, the fine crepitation and thickening indicative of tenosynovitis may be felt. It is helpful for the examiner to place only one of his fingers across the palmar aspect of the metacarpal heads to avoid affecting the patient's ability to make a fist. The patient then actively flexes the metacarpophalangeal joints as far as possible before flexing the proximal and distal interphalangeal joints. This procedure produces a maximal excursion of the flexor tendons and enables the examiner to palpate for crepitation while the tendons move throughout their range of motion. "Rice bodies" or fibrin clumps that give a feeling described as that of "lead shot in a leather bag" may be found by palpation in the presence of some types of chronic tenosynovitis. Sometimes localized cystic outpouchings of the tendon synovial sheaths may be palpated in the palm.

Palpation of the palmar aspect of the hand may reveal nodular enlargement of one or more of the flexor tendons. This almost always occurs at the level of the metacarpal head, where a reinforcement or thickening of the deep fascia forms a proximal annular ligament in the sheath of the flexor tendon; this area of thickening is referred to as the "proximal pulley." A finger in which such an enlargement has developed may become temporarily or even persistently locked in the position of flexion or extension when the tendon is unable to move normally because of the nodular enlargement, stenosis of the tendon sheath, or both, at the level of the proximal pulley. When additional force is applied and the finger can be moved beyond its fixed position, the nodular enlargement may be pulled through the constricted area, suddenly releasing or snapping the finger into the limit of the range of either extension or flexion, whichever was restricted previously. A click or snap may be felt (and sometimes heard) as the nodular enlargement of the tendon is actively moved past the area of constriction in the tendon sheath. This condition is known as a "trigger" or "snapping" digit. Locking usually occurs when the affected finger is in flexion. Tenderness over the proximal pulley, especially in the thumb, is suggestive of tenosynovitis of the flexor tendons before locking occurs. Although the flexors of the fingers and thumb are stronger than the extensors, the absence of a tendon sheath on the extensor tendons and the presence of a tendon sheath (which may become inflamed, thickened, or stenosed) on the flexor tendons are probably more significant factors than is the comparative strength of the tendons. A trigger or snapping digit involves the first (thumb) and fourth (ring) fingers most frequently but may involve any finger. In patients with rheumatoid arthritis the third (middle) and fourth (ring) fingers are involved more often than the other digits.

Palmar Fascia. This should be palpated for the presence of fibrous bands and nodules, which are to be differentiated from nodular enlargements of flexor tendons. Such palmar nodules are found most often near the distal palmar crease of the fourth digit, but they also may involve the region of the palm near the fifth and third digits. The skin is often irregularly attached over the involved area (Dupuytren's contracture; Fig. 9–9).

Special tests for specific conditions will be considered later in this chapter.

MOVEMENT AND RANGE OF MOTION

Movements of the wrist include palmar flexion (flexion), dorsiflexion (extension), radial deviation, and ulnar deviation. A combination of these movements allows circumduction of the wrist. These movements require varying degrees of motion at both the radiocarpal and the midcarpal joints. Limited flexion and extension and slight rotation are permitted in the midcarpal joint. Pronation and supination of the hand and forearm occur primarily at the proximal and distal radio-ulnar articulations.

The carpometacarpal joints move very little, with the exception of the carpometacarpal joint of the thumb, which possesses the movements of a ball-and-socket joint (flexion, extension, adduction, abduction, and medial and lateral rotation) and which is set at an angle so that flexion and abduction bring the thumb into apposition with the fingers.

The range of wrist motion varies considerably among different individuals and is best evaluated when the examiner grasps the patient's forearm proximal to the wrist and allows the patient to demonstrate range of motion actively. Comparison of motion of the two wrists should be made with both wrists and hands in the same position. It is preferable to examine motion of the wrist with the patient's hand and forearm in pronation since supination and pronation of the hand and forearm influence motion.

Measurements of range of motion in the wrist should start with the wrist and hand in a straight position in relation to the forearm (0 degrees). The wrist usually can be dorsiflexed about 70 degrees and palmar flexed about 80 to 90 degrees from the straight position (Fig. 9–15). Ulnar deviation averages about 50 to 60 degrees from the straight position and exceeds radial deviation, which averages about 20 degrees. Loss or limitation of dorsiflexion is the most common and important functional impairment of wrist motion.

MUSCLE TESTING

Flexion. The prime movers in flexion of the wrist are the flexor carpi radialis (median nerve, C6, 7) and the flexor carpi ulnaris (ulnar nerve, C8, T1) muscles. The palmaris longus muscle is accessory to this motion. Flexion is tested while the patient sits with his forearm supinated and resting comfortably on a table, which helps to stabilize it. The muscles of the thumb and other fingers should be relaxed. The examiner holds the patient's forearm in the middle with one hand for further stabilization while the patient flexes the wrist against graded resistance provided by the fingertips of the examiner's other hand placed in the patient's palm. The flexor carpi radialis muscle is tested when the examiner provides resistance on the palmar side of the base of the second metacar-

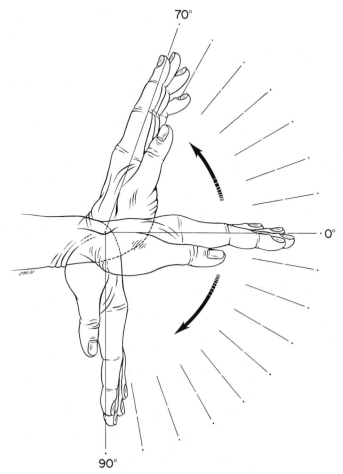

70°

0°

90°

Figure 9–15. Range of normal flexion and extension of the wrist.

pal bone in the directions of extension and ulnar deviation, as shown in Figure 9–16. The flexor carpi ulnaris is tested when the examiner applies resistance on the palmar side of the base of the fifth metacarpal bone in the directions of extension and radial deviation.

Extension. The prime movers in extension of the wrist are the extensor carpi radialis longus (radial nerve, C6, 7), extensor carpi radialis brevis (radial nerve, C6, 7), and extensor carpi ulnaris (radial nerve, C7, 8) muscles. Extension is tested while the patient sits with the pronated forearm resting on a table. The muscles of the thumb and other fingers should be relaxed. The examiner holds the patient's forearm in the middle with one hand to stabilize it while the patient extends the wrist against graded resistance applied by the examiner's other hand to the dorsal surface of the patient's metacarpals. For testing the extensor carpi radialis longus and brevis muscles, resistance is applied by the ex-

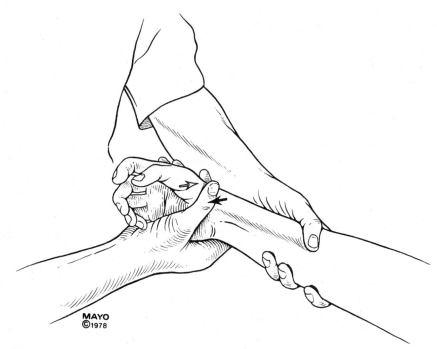

MAYO
©1978

Figure 9–16. Test for the flexor carpi radialis. With fingers relaxed, the patient flexes the wrist. The examiner stabilizes the forearm with one hand and with the other hand resists flexion in the direction of extension and ulnar deviation.

aminer to the dorsal surface of the second and third metacarpal bones in the directions of flexion and ulnar deviation. For testing the extensor carpi ulnaris muscle, resistance is applied to the dorsal surface of the fifth metacarpal bone in the directions of flexion and radial deviation. When the forearm is pronated, the extensor carpi ulnaris muscle lies lateral to the ulnar head and acts as a strong ulnar deviator.

Supination of Forearm.   The prime movers in supination of the forearm are the biceps brachii (musculocutaneous nerve, C5, 6) and supinator (radial nerve, C6) muscles; the brachioradialis muscle is accessory to this motion. Supination is tested while the patient sits with the arm at his side, the elbow flexed to 90 degrees to prevent rotation at the shoulder, and the forearm pronated. Muscles of the wrists and fingers should be relaxed. The examiner grasps and holds the arm with one hand to stabilize it. The patient then supinates the forearm against graded resistance provided by the examiner's other hand at the distal end of the radius.

Pronation of Forearm.   The prime movers in pronation of the forearm are the pronator teres (median nerve, C6, 7) and the pronator quadratus (palmar interosseous branch of the median nerve, C8, T1). The flexor carpi radialis muscle is accessory to this motion. Pronation is tested with the patient's arm at his side, elbow flexed to 90 degrees, and

forearm supinated. The muscles of the wrist and fingers should be relaxed. The examiner stabilizes the patient's arm with one hand. The patient then pronates the forearm through the range of motion against
graded resistance provided by the examiner's other hand at the distal end
of the radius.

SPECIAL TESTS FOR INVOLVEMENT OF
STRUCTURES NEAR THE WRIST

Carpometacarpal Joint of the First Digit

The carpometacarpal joint of the thumb is a relatively common
site for the changes of degenerative joint disease, and sometimes bony
spurs and crepitation may be felt at the base of the thumb when this
joint is involved. Tenderness or swelling or both at the base of the
thumb (carpometacarpal joint) should be differentiated from that resulting from involvement of the wrist. The carpometacarpal joint of the
thumb can be further evaluated by the following two maneuvers:

1. While the muscles of the patient's thumb are relaxed to avoid
symptoms due to muscle spasm or tender muscle attachments, the examiner grasps the thumb near the metacarpophalangeal joint and firmly
pushes the thumb inward toward the carpometacarpal joint. This maneuver often produces pain in the region of the carpometacarpal joint if
disease of this joint is present.

2. Crepitation of the carpometacarpal joint of the thumb is best
palpated at the base of the thumb with the fingers of one of the examiner's hands, while the fingers of the examiner's other hand grasp the patient's thumb in the region of the proximal phalanx and move it in a
clockwise rotation.

Stenosing Tenosynovitis at the Radial
Styloid Process (de Quervain's
Tenosynovitis)

This condition characteristically involves both the long abductor
and short extensor tendons of the thumb (de Quervain's tenosynovitis;
Fig. 9–4). Tenderness near the radial styloid process can be localized
further by having the patient place his thumb in the palm of his hand and
flex his fingers over the thumb. The patient's hand should be held loosely in this position. If there is no accentuation of the pain or tenderness
with the thumb in this position, the examiner grasps the patient's hand
and cautiously moves the patient's wrist into ulnar deviation. This maneuver may cause severe pain over the radial styloid process when the
test is positive because of the extra tension on the long abductor tendon

of the thumb and should be performed with caution when stenosing ten-osynovitis is suspected. Comparison with the same maneuver on the op-posite side helps one evaluate the patient's reactions.

Compression of the Median Nerve in the Carpal Tunnel (Carpal Tunnel Syndrome)

The carpal tunnel syndrome usually is caused by thickening of the synovial membrane about the flexor tendons. The presence of tenosyn-ovitis often can be observed by inspection when the flexor aspect of the wrist is tangential to the examiner's eyes or can be felt during palpation.

When the wrist is maintained in acute palmar flexion for 60 sec-onds, numbness and paresthesia often occur in the hand and fingers over the distribution of the median nerve, especially on the palmar surface of the first three digits and a portion of the fourth digit (Phalen's sign). These symptoms are relieved within a few minutes after the wrist as-sumes a straight position. Sometimes acute extension of the wrist will produce similar symptoms and should be tried when acute palmar flexion of the wrist does not aggravate median nerve compression. Symptoms also can be produced by placing a blood pressure cuff on the upper arm and inflating it above the level of systolic blood pressure for 3 to 5 min-utes. Percussion of the volar aspect of the wrist over the median nerve may be performed to determine whether a tingling or prickling sensation results in the hand over the distribution of the median nerve. The tin-gling or prickling, when present, suggests compression of the median nerve (Tinel's sign), but it also can occur in individuals without true com-pression of the median nerve. Decreased sweating on the flexor surface of the digits supplied by the median nerve can be detected in some pa-tients with the carpal tunnel syndrome.

Since the flexor pollicis longus, the abductor pollicis brevis, and the opponens pollicis muscles are supplied by the median nerve, they are often weakened when the median nerve is chronically compressed. These muscles, therefore, should be tested when the carpal tunnel syndrome is suspected (see p. 144). Atrophy of the thenar muscles may occur with prolonged median nerve compression (Fig. 9–10) and is detected by tests described in Chapter 10. Confirmation of weakness and atrophy due to median nerve compression is obtained by electromyographic measure-ments of the conduction time of the median nerve.

Marfan's Syndrome

The arachnodactyly of Marfan's syndrome often results in a com-bination of elongated digits and a forearm that is of small circumference near the wrist. When such a patient grasps with one hand the wrist of the other hand about 4 cm proximal to the radial or ulnar styloid process, fingers 1 and 5 of the grasping hand overlap appreciably (wrist sign described by Walker and Murdoch).

Another test of arachnodactyly and the laxity of capsules, ligaments, and tendons found in Marfan's syndrome involves having the patient make a fist with the thumb inside the flexed fingers (that is, opposed across the palm). In such patients and in a very small percentage of children without Marfan's syndrome, the distal portion of the thumb extends well beyond the ulnar margin of the hand (thumb sign described by Steinberg).

Camptodactyly (fixation of a digit in flexion) of the fifth finger is another possible physical finding in Marfan's syndrome.

SUGGESTED READING FOR ADDITIONAL INFORMATION

1. Flatt AE: The Care of the Rheumatoid Hand. Third edition. St. Louis, CV Mosby Company, 1974, 296 pp.
2. Boyes JH: Bunnell's Surgery of the Hand. Fifth edition. Philadelphia, JB Lippincott Company, 1970, 727 pp. (Chapters 1, 4, 9, and 12.)
3. Cailliet R: Hand Pain and Impairment. Second edition. Philadelphia, FA Davis Company, 1975, 170 pp.
4. Landsmeer JMF: Atlas of Anatomy of the Hand. Edinburgh, Churchill Livingstone, 1976, 349 pp.
5. Lipman BS, Massie E: Clubbed fingers and hypertrophic osteoarthropathy. In: MacBryde CM, Blacklow RS (editors): Signs and Symptoms: Applied Pathologic Physiology and Clinical Interpretation. Fifth edition. Philadelphia, JB Lippincott Company, 1970, pp. 256–271.
6. Cracchiolo III A: The carpal tunnel syndrome. Semin Arthritis Rheum 1:87–95, 1971.

chapter **10**

The Metacarpophalangeal, Proximal and Distal Interphalangeal Joints

ESSENTIAL ANATOMY

Joints, Ligaments, and Tendons

    Metacarpophalangeal Joints. These joints (which usually are considered hinge joints) have dense fibrous or fibrocartilaginous ligaments over the palmar surface (known as the volar plate) and are reinforced by collateral ligaments on each side. These collateral ligaments, which become tight in flexion and loose in extension, prevent lateral motion of the digit distal to the metacarpophalangeal joint when it is flexed.

112

An extensor tendon crosses the dorsum of each joint and strengthens the thin articular capsule in this region. When the extensor tendon of the digit reaches the distal end of the metacarpal head, it is joined by fibers of the interossei and lumbricales and thus expands over the entire dorsum of the metacarpophalangeal joint and onto the dorsum of the adjacent phalanx. This expansion of the extensor mechanism is known as the extensor hood. Opposite the metacarpophalangeal joint each extensor tendon is bound by fasciculi to the collateral ligaments. (The anatomy of the flexor tendons of the hand is discussed in Chapter 9.)

Proximal and Distal Interphalangeal Joints.   The proximal and distal interphalangeal joints are similar anatomically. They are true hinge joints whose movements are restricted to flexion and extension. The ligaments of the interphalangeal joints resemble those of the metacarpophalangeal joints. Each interphalangeal joint has a thin dorsal capsular ligament strengthened by expansion of the extensor tendon, a dense palmar ligament (volar plate), and collateral ligaments that strengthen each side of the joint. Opposite the proximal interphalangeal joint the extensor tendon divides into three slips: one intermediate and two collateral. The intermediate slip is inserted into the base of the second phalanx, and the two collateral slips extend along the sides of the second phalanx to unite and insert into the dorsal surface of the terminal phalanx. The palmar and collateral ligaments normally help prevent hyperextension of the proximal and distal interphalangeal joints.

Articular Capsule and Synovial Membrane

When the fingers are flexed, the heads of the metacarpal bones form the rounded prominences of the knuckles, with the metacarpophalangeal joint spaces lying about 1 cm distal to the apices of these prominences (Fig. 10–1). The distal part of the articular capsule and the synovial membrane that lines the inner surface of the capsule are both attached firmly to the base of the proximal phalanx and the metacarpal head, but the articular capsule is loose over the metacarpal head (Figs. 9–1 and 9–2). Figure 9–1 shows the relationship of the dorsal aspect of the joint space, the synovial membrane, and the articular capsule to adjacent and overlying structures. The skin on the palmar surface of the hand is relatively thick and covers a fat pad between it and the metacarpophalangeal joint; this makes palpation of the palmar surface of the joint space and articular capsule more difficult and less satisfactory than palpation of the dorsolateral surfaces.

The distribution of the articular capsule and synovial membrane of the proximal and distal interphalangeal joints is similar to that of the metacarpophalangeal joint. Both the synovial membrane and the articular capsule of the interphalangeal joints are firmly attached distally to the base of the more distal phalanx forming the joint and firmly but more

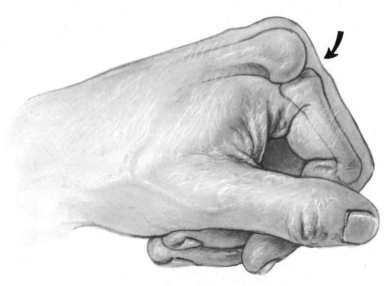

Figure 10–1. Schematic diagram of medial aspect of hand. Arrow indicates that the metacarpophalangeal joint space lies distal to the prominence of the knuckle when the proximal phalanx is flexed on the metacarpophalangeal joint.

extensively to the phalanx forming the proximal portion of the joint (Fig. 9–2).

INSPECTION

Swelling of the metacarpophalangeal and interphalangeal joints may result from articular or periarticular causes. The loss of normal knuckle wrinkles is indicative of soft-tissue swelling and suggests synovitis of the involved joints if the swelling is restricted to the distribution of the synovial membrane and articular capsule. Synovial swelling (Figs. 10–2 and 10–3) produces symmetric enlargement of the joint, whereas extra-articular swelling (Figs. 10–4 and 10–5) may be diffuse and is often asymmetric, involving one side of the joint but not the other. This differentiation is exemplified by comparison of Figures 10–2 and 10–4; Figure 10–2 shows synovitis in the metacarpophalangeal joints, while Figure 10–4 shows diffuse edema on the dorsum of the hands and in the region of the metacarpophalangeal joints.

Synovial distention or thickening of a metacarpophalangeal joint may produce stretching and eventual relaxation of the articular capsule and ligaments. This combined with muscle imbalance and the force of gravity may cause the extensor tendon of the digit to slip off the metacarpal head on the ulnar side of the joint. The abnormal pull of the tendon resulting from this displacement may contribute significantly to the development of an ulnar deviation or "drift" of the fingers (Figs.

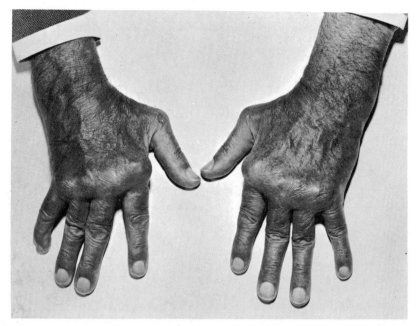

Figure 10–2. Characteristic soft-tissue swelling (synovitis, grade 2) and flexion contractures of the metacarpophalangeal joints and hyperextension of proximal interphalangeal joints of second to fifth digits, inclusive, in a patient with advanced rheumatoid arthritis. Ulnar deviation of the fingers is especially evident in patient's right hand. Muscular atrophy of hands, synovitis of wrists, and radial deviation of the carpometacarpal unit of the hands are also present.

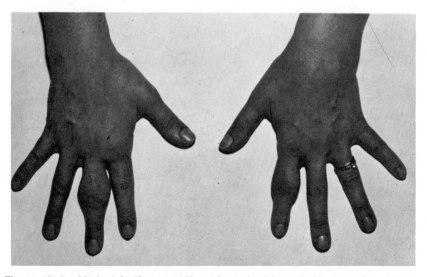

Figure 10–3. Marked fusiform swelling of proximal interphalangeal joints of third digit in right hand (synovitis, grade 4) and second digit in left hand (synovitis, grade 3) in patient with rheumatoid arthritis. Fusiform swelling of the proximal interphalangeal joints commonly occurs in rheumatoid arthritis, but it is more characteristically symmetric than is the asymmetric involvement of the fingers shown here.

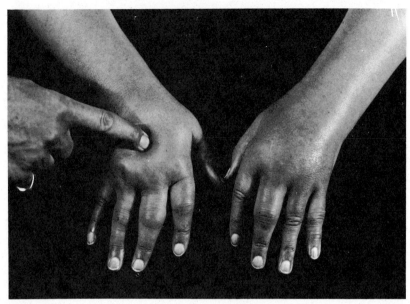

Figure 10–4. Massive diffuse edema of both hands associated with but obscuring synovitis of the wrists and metacarpophalangeal joints. The swelling in the proximal interphalangeal joints, especially evident in the third finger of each hand, is in the distribution of the synovial membrane and can be differentiated on palpation from the edema extending into the area of the proximal phalanx from the dorsum of the hand. Patient had rheumatoid arthritis.

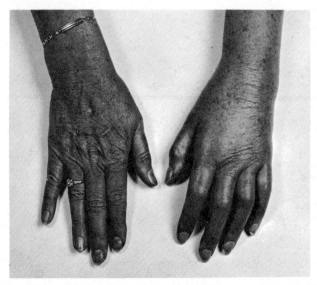

Figure 10–5. Diffuse edema and swelling in left hand (associated with limitation of left shoulder) in established shoulder-hand syndrome.

10–2, 10–6, and 10–7). However, ulnar deviation results from multiple factors, which may vary in different instances. When ulnar deviation of the fingers occurs, subluxation of one or more proximal phalanges of the fingers at the metacarpophalangeal joint or joints often is associated.

Hyperextension of the proximal interphalangeal joints results when the interossei or the lateral expansion of the extensor mechanism becomes thickened and shortened or the extensor tendon is pushed dorsally by the distended joint capsule. In the hyperextended position, flexion of the interphalangeal joints is difficult for the patient to initiate. Hyperextension of the proximal interphalangeal joint is often associated with partial flexion of the distal interphalangeal joint due to tightening of the flexor tendon to the terminal phalanx.

The term "swan-neck deformity" is used to describe the appearance of a finger resulting from contracture of the interossei and flexor muscles or tendons that produces a flexion contracture of the metacarpophalangeal joint, sequential hyperextension of the proximal interphalangeal joint, and flexion of the distal interphalangeal joint (Fig. 10–8). The term "swan-neck deformity" was suggested because the contracture resembles the curved shape of a swan's neck. A similar deformity characterized by flexion of the metacarpophalangeal joint and hyperextension of the interphalangeal joint may occur in the thumb. Such swan-neck contractures often are accompanied by ulnar drift of the fingers.

When a swan-neck deformity is present, the patient is unable to

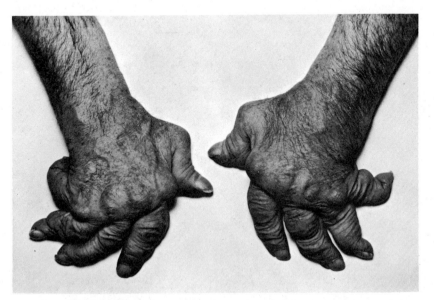

Figure 10–6. Severe deformities of both hands in patient with advanced rheumatoid arthritis. There is chronic synovitis and subluxation of metacarpophalangeal joints, marked ulnar deviation of fingers, shortening of digits and wrinkling of skin over damaged joints, producing the opera-glass hand or "la main en lorgnette."

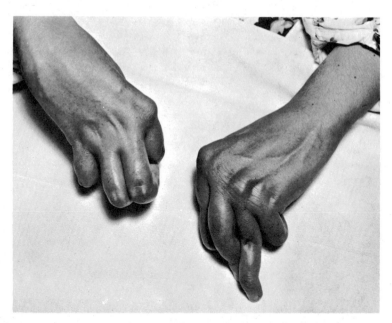

Figure 10–7.   Another type of severe deformity of the fingers in a patient with rheumatoid arthritis. The right wrist is swollen and ankylosed in mild flexion. The metacarpophalangeal joints of the third, fourth, and fifth digits on the right are hyperextended and there are flexion contractures of the proximal interphalangeal joints of these digits. The metacarpophalangeal joints of the left hand are flexed, the proximal interphalangeal joints of the second and fourth digits are hyperextended, and the distal interphalangeal joints in the same digits are flexed (swan-neck deformity). The proximal interphalangeal joints of the left third and fifth digits are flexed, the distal interphalangeal joints of the left third digit is hyperextended and that of the fifth digit is flexed but not fully visualized in this photograph. Ulnar deviation is present in both hands but is more marked on the left.

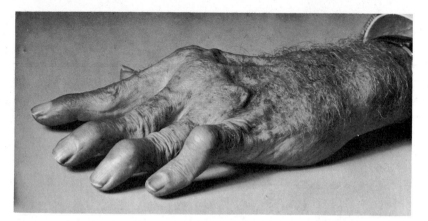

Figure 10–8.   Flexion of the metacarpophalangeal joints, hyperextension of the proximal interphalangeal joints and flexion of distal interphalangeal joints in the second, third, and fourth digits in patient with rheumatoid arthritis ("intrinsic-plus" or "swan-neck" deformity). In the fifth digit the proximal interphalangeal joint is flexed and the distal interphalangeal joint hyperextended (boutonnière deformity).

flex the proximal interphalangeal joint while the metacarpophalangeal joint of the affected digit (or digits) is held in extension because the intrinsic muscles are elongated over both the metacarpophalangeal and the proximal interphalangeal joints by this motion. When it is noted that the proximal interphalangeal joints cannot be actively flexed in this position, the examiner should passively flex all three of the joints of the digit to determine whether the limitation of interphalangeal flexion results from the swan-neck deformity, from destructive disease of the joint, or from involvement of the extensor tendons.

In the normal hand there is a balance between the pull exerted by the long flexors, the long extensors, and the intrinsic muscles. When the intrinsic muscles and their tendons exert an "overpull," the hand develops "intrinsic-plus" contractures such as the "swan-neck" deformity just described. If the intrinsic muscles are paralyzed by loss of innervation from both the median and ulnar nerves, the hand assumes an "intrinsic-minus" position usually referred to as a paralytic or "claw" hand. A claw hand is characterized by hyperextension of the metacarpophalangeal joints, flexion of the proximal and distal interphalangeal joints, flattening or loss of the metacarpal arch, and adduction and external rotation of the thumb.

The term "boutonnière deformity" is used to describe flexion of the proximal interphalangeal joint accompanied by compensatory hyperextension of the distal interphalangeal joint of the same digit (Fig. 10–8). This relatively common deformity results from detachment of the central slip of the extensor tendon of the proximal interphalangeal joint from the base of the middle phalanx, which thus allows dislocation of the lateral bands in a palmar direction. When the dislocated lateral bands cross the fulcrum of the joint, they act as flexors instead of extensors of the joint. As a result of this distortion, the proximal and distal phalanges of the joint are pushed between the two dislocated lateral bands. The anatomic appearance is that of a knuckle being pushed through a buttonhole, hence the derivation of the term "boutonnière deformity." Occasionally in the presence of tenosynovitis of flexor tendons, the affected tendon will sublux away from the volar aspect of the joint, thus increasing greatly the mechanical advantage of the tendon and producing a "secondary boutonnière deformity."

Helpful information is obtained from recognition of abnormalities of the terminal digits, including bony, soft-tissue, and nail changes. Bony changes may be evident as osteophytic articular nodules. When these occur on the distal interphalangeal joints they are described as Heberden's nodes and when on the proximal interphalangeal joints as Bouchard's nodes (Fig. 10–9); similar nodules result from trauma, infection, or chronic inflammation. Telescopic shortening of the digits produced by resorption of the ends of the phalanges is associated with wrinkling of the skin over the involved joints (opera-glass hand or "la main en lorgnette," Fig. 10–6).

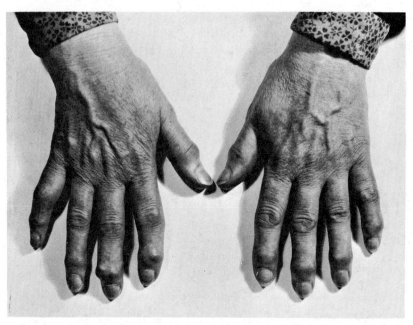

Figure 10–9. Degenerative joint disease (osteoarthritis) of both hands. Osteoarthritic enlargement of the distal interphalangeal joints (Heberden's nodes) and the proximal interphalangeal joints (Bouchard's nodes) is present. The metacapophalangeal joints are not affected.

Soft-tissue changes include synovial cysts on the dorsolateral aspects of the joints (Fig. 10–10), thickening of the fibrous capsule that produces an extra-articular swelling on the dorsum of the proximal interphalangeal joints ("dorsal knuckle pads"; Fig. 10–11), and clubbing of the terminal phalanges (Figs. 10–12 and 10–13). When clubbing is in advanced stages, it may be associated with hypertrophic osteoarthropathy. The term "pulmonary periostopathy" has been proposed* as more descriptive. The condition, however, is not limited to disorders of pulmonary origin.

Other soft-tissue changes in the hands include the presence of soft-tissue nodules or urate tophi (Fig. 10–14). Nail changes include pitting, ridging, thickening, discoloration (Fig. 10–15), or watch-crystal rounding (Fig. 10–12). The latter is sometimes associated with clubbing of the terminal phalanx. The presence of clubbing is recognized by obliteration of the normal angle (about 160 degrees) at the base of the nail and in advanced stages by upward projection of the base of the nail (positive profile sign). Observation of the angle or of its obliteration is often enhanced when the distal interphalangeal joint is partially flexed (Fig. 10–13). Changes in the skin include pallor, rubor, edema, atrophy, ulcers and hidebound tightening. Figures 10–16 through 10–22 give examples of types of conditions visible on inspection.

---

*JAMA *194*:546, 1965.

Text continued on page 128

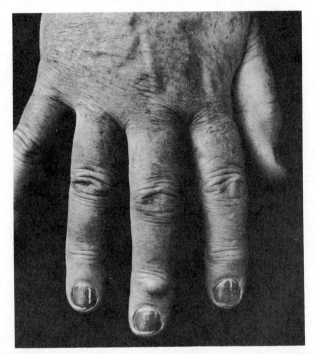

Figure 10–10. Synovial cyst from distal interphalangeal joint of third digit of a patient with Heberden's nodes.

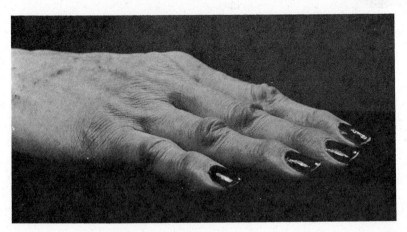

Figure 10–11. Thickening and elevation of skin and subcutaneous tissues on dorsal aspect of proximal interphalangeal joints without evidence of arthritis. This condition is known as "dorsal knuckle pads."

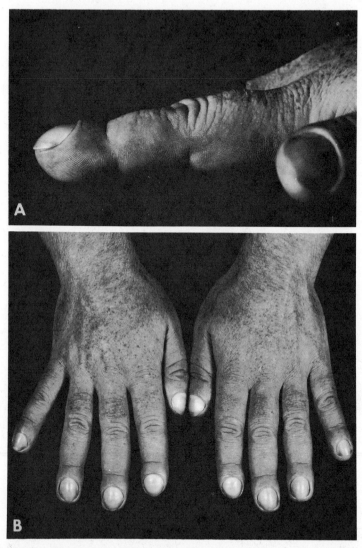

Figure 10–12. Clubbing of distal interphalangeal joints and rounding of the nails in a patient with hypertrophic osteoarthropathy. *A.* Close up, side view of second (index) finger. *B.* Dorsal aspect of both hands.

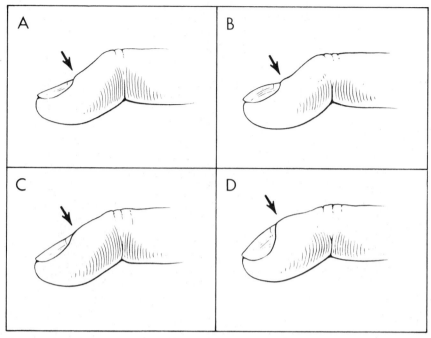

Figure 10–13. Profiles of distal phalanx of a finger. *A.* Normal finger illustrating the normal angle at the base of the fingernail (usually about 160 degrees). *B.* Variant of normal showing curving of the nail. The normal angle at the base of the nail is retained. *C.* Early clubbing with obliteration of the angle at the base of the nail. *D.* Advanced clubbing. The angle at the base of the nail is greater than 180 degrees and the base of the nail projects upward.

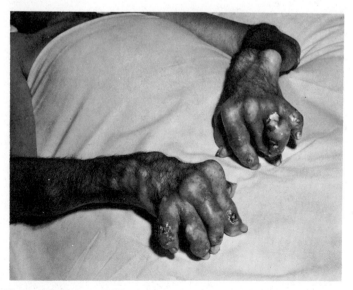

Figure 10–14. Multiple tophi in forearms, wrists, and hands with ulceration and drainage of urates from tophi in several proximal and distal interphalangeal joints of a patient with severe chronic gouty arthritis. Modern treatment has made such extensive changes rare.

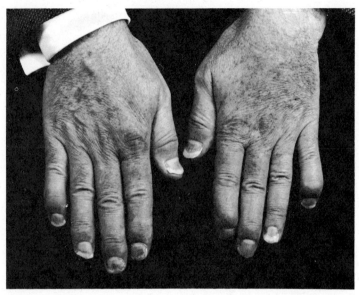

Figure 10–15. Swelling and flexion of several distal interphalangeal joints and pitting, discoloration, and elevation of terminal portion of nails in a patient with psoriatic arthritis.

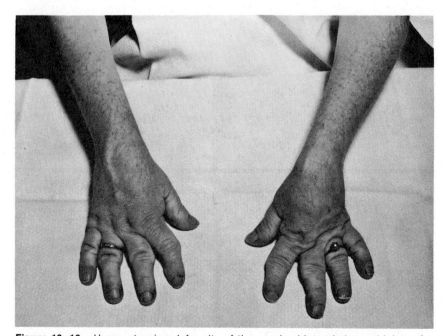

Figure 10–16. Hyperextension deformity of the proximal interphalangeal joints of a patient whose rheumatoid arthritis had a juvenile onset and was associated with stunting of growth. Arthropathic resorption of phalanges and articulations resulted in wrinkling and redundancy of the skin of the digits and hypermobility of meta-carpophalangeal and proximal interphalangeal joints. This photograph also shows synovial swelling of both wrists. The patient also had limited motion of these joints.

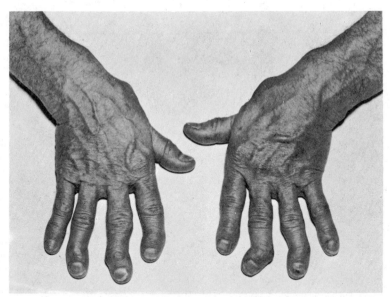

Figure 10–17. Deviation of the distal phalanx at the distal interphalangeal joint in the second, third, and fourth digits of the right hand and in the third and fourth digits of the left hand in a patient with degenerative joint disease (osteoarthritis). Heberden's nodes are seen at the distal interphalangeal joints, some bony enlargement is present in the proximal interphalangeal joints, and there is a bony prominence of the carpometacarpal joint at the base of each thumb. The ulnar deviation of the first metacarpal bone is characteristic of degenerative joint disease of the first carpometacarpal joint.

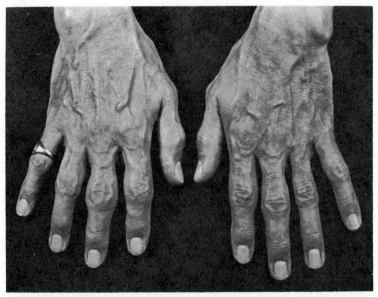

Figure 10–18. Degenerative joint disease (osteoarthritis) of both hands. Bony enlargement of proximal interphalangeal joints, Heberden's nodes in distal interphalangeal joints, and characteristic sparing of the metacarpophalangeal joints should be noted.

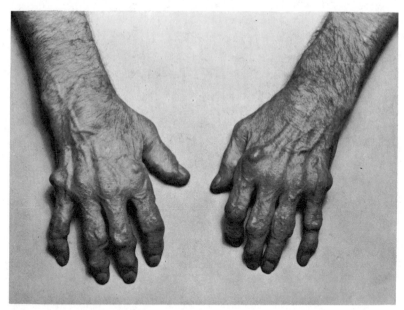

Figure 10–19. Multiple firm subcutaneous nodules in both hands of a patient with rheumatoid arthritis.

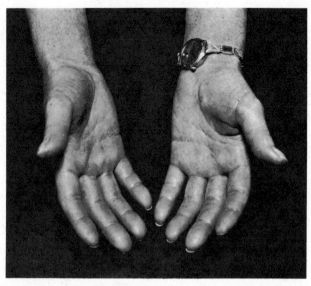

Figure 10–20. Diffuse puffiness of fingers but no atrophy or contractures in a patient with scleroderma and early acrosclerosis.

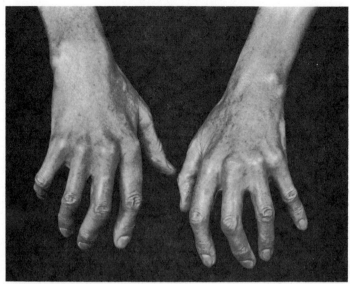

Figure 10–21.   Tight, shiny, hidebound, atrophic skin and flexion deformities at the proximal interphalangeal joints in a stage of scleroderma with acrosclerosis more advanced than in Figure 10–20.

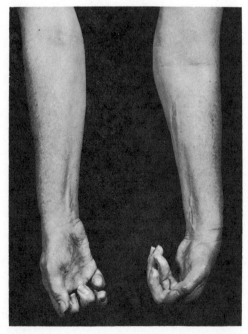

Figure 10–22.   Palmar fascial atrophy and contractures and flexion deformities of fingers of both hands in the late (residual) stage of bilateral shoulder-hand syndrome.

PALPATION

Metacarpophalangeal Joints

The metacarpophalangeal joint is palpated for evidence of synovial thickening or distention, tenderness, and warmth in three locations: in the region of the joint space, over the metacarpal head, and in the groove between adjacent metacarpal heads. Normally the synovial membrane cannot be palpated in the region of the joint space, but in the presence of synovial thickening the bony margins of the joint space are obscured by swelling. The joint space is felt most easily about 1 cm distal to the apex of the knuckles (Fig. 10–1) with the proximal phalanx flexed about 20 to 30 degrees on the metacarpophalangeal joint. It is palpated best over the dorsolateral aspects of the joint on each side of the extensor tendon (Fig. 10–23).

The extensor tendon of the digit can be delineated easily in the midline as it crosses the dorsum of the joint, but adequate examination of the portion of the joint directly beneath this structure is not possible under normal conditions. Distention of the synovial membrane and articular capsule, however, may cause stretching and eventual relaxation of the articular capsule and ligaments, so that the extensor tendon of the

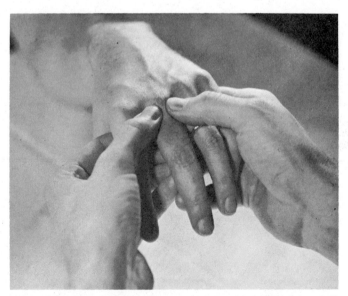

Figure 10–23. Palpation of third metacarpophalangeal joint of left hand. Examiner's thumbs are palpating dorsal aspect of joint while forefingers (not seen in this photograph) are palpating volar aspect of metacarpal head. The joint being examined is held in a relaxed position of partial flexion. The examiner's remaining fingers support the patient's hand. The other metacarpophalangeal joints are similarly examined. Compare with Figure 10–1 showing the position of the joint relative to the prominence of the knuckle.

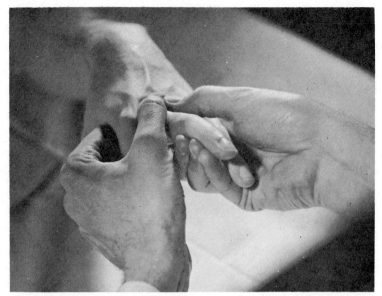

Figure 10–24. Alternate position for palpation over dorsal aspect of metacarpo-phalangeal joints. The palpating thumbs are proximal to the level of the joint line (see Fig. 10–1). The joint is examined in a position midway between hyperextension and dorsiflexion or in slight hyperextension, as shown here. The position and function of the examiner's digits are similar to those shown and described in Figure 10–23.

digit is allowed to slip off the prominence of the metacarpal head. When this occurs, the tendon can be palpated on the ulnar side of the metacarpal head in the longitudinal groove between adjacent metacarpal heads, and then the exposed joint space can be palpated easily over the dorsal aspect of the joint.

The region of the joint space is palpated with the joint partially flexed, and then the metacarpal head and joint space also are palpated with the joint extended. The finger of the metacarpophalangeal joint being examined is held in extension by the examiner's fingers during the examination, as this relaxes the articular capsule and enables the examiner to feel synovial thickening more easily (Fig. 10–24). Extension of the metacarpophalangeal joint accentuates any soft-tissue swelling of synovitis but also may cause distention of periarticular tissues. Such distention then needs to be differentiated from synovial swelling.

The region over the metacarpal head and the longitudinal groove between adjacent metacarpal heads also are palpated for evidence of synovial thickening or distention. Normally the synovial membrane cannot be palpated in this groove, but in the presence of synovial thickening or distention the groove on both sides of the involved joint, the normal hard bony landmarks of the metacarpal heads, and the joint spaces are obliterated. Synovial thickening can be evaluated more completely by rolling the palpating thumb and finger or both thumbs over the dorsolateral aspects of the metacarpal heads (Fig. 10–25). Interpretation of the examination findings would be facilitated by again referring to the anatomy and the attachments of the synovial membrane described in the "Anatomy" section of this chapter and shown in Figure 10–1. The soft-tissue swelling of synovitis is symmetric in relation to the involved joint and may be associated with warmth and tenderness. If soft-tissue swelling is present only on one side of a metacarpal head, it most likely lies outside the articular capsule and is not due to an intra-articular reaction.

To palpate the metacarpophalangeal joint, the patient's hand should be relaxed and in as comfortable a position as possible with the palm turned down and the wrist in pronation. Each joint is examined separately by grasping the joint firmly between both of the examiner's thumbs, which are placed on the dorsum of the joint, and both index fingers, which are placed on the palmar aspect of the joint, while the examiner's remaining fingers support the patient's hand (Fig. 10–23). In an alternative method, the examiner palpates the dorsal aspect of the joint between the thumb and index finger of one hand while his other hand supports the patient's hand. With either method, examination of the metacarpophalangeal joint should include palpation of the joint space, the metacarpal head, and the longitudinal groove between adjacent metacarpal heads for evidence of synovial thickening or distention with

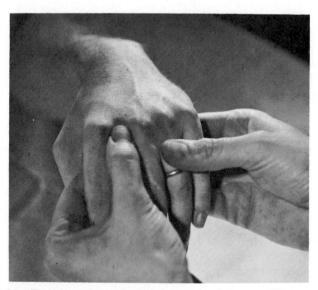

Figure 10–25. Technique for palpation in groove between adjacent metacarpal heads of left hand for evidence of synovial or other swelling. The left thumb of the examiner is palpating deeply. It is alternately turned to feel each adjacent metacarpal head and joint. The examiner's right hand and the digits of the left hand not being used in palpation support the patient's hand. For assessment of synovial swelling, the technique shown in Figures 10–23 and 10–24, using both thumbs simultaneously, is more accurate. See text for details.

the joint flexed and also with the joint extended (Figs. 10–23, 10–24, and 10–25).

The examiner's index fingers, when placed on the palmar surface of the metacarpal head, should feel for tenderness and fullness while the joint is compressed between the examiner's thumbs on the dorsal surface and the index fingers. Subluxation of the proximal phalanx on the metacarpal head may occur toward the palmar aspect of the hand; when this happens, the bony landmarks of the adjacent phalanx are more prominent than they are normally.

If an "intrinsic-plus" muscle contracture is present, the metacarpophalangeal joint cannot be extended fully, and when full extension is attempted passively, the proximal interphalangeal joint goes into hyperextension and the distal interphalangeal joint into flexion, producing the swan-neck deformity of the digit. If this condition is accompanied by ulnar drift of the fingers, the contractures are accentuated when the examiner passively moves the digit toward the radial side of the hand to bring the finger back to its realigned straight position in relationship to its metacarpal.

Proximal Interphalangeal Joints

In palpation of the proximal interphalangeal joint, the soft-tissue swelling of knuckle pads on the dorsal aspect and tenosynovial reactions of flexor tendon sheaths must be distinguished from true synovial reactions involving the joint. Synovial swelling indicates a reaction throughout the synovial membrane; local tenderness, warmth, or redness may or may not be associated. Swelling is most readily palpable on the medial and lateral aspects of the joint and just proximal to the joint space because of the looser and more extensive attachment of the synovial membrane to the proximal phalanx as compared to the middle phalanx and because an expansion of the extensor tendon of the digit covers the dorsum of the proximal interphalangeal joint. The soft-tissue swelling of tenosynovitis usually involves the palmar aspect of the joint and may be associated with tenderness, local warmth, induration, and locking or crepitation when motion of the digit is attempted. Thickening of the skin and subcutaneous tissue over the dorsal aspect of the proximal interphalangeal joints (knuckle pad) appears as localized, superficial, nontender swelling without local heat or redness but with a firmer consistency than that of synovial distention and should not be confused with swelling in the distribution of the synovial membrane or joint capsule.

When diffuse swelling of the digits occurs, it extends over the region of the joint as well as between the joints. It is difficult or impossible to palpate through this swelling to evaluate intra-articular synovial reactions. Palpable bony enlargement of articular margins can be differentiated without difficulty from the "boggy" soft-tissue reaction of synovial swelling.

In palpation of the proximal interphalangeal joint, the examiner supports the patient's hand with one hand while palpating each proximal interphalangeal joint between the thumb and index finger of his other hand placed on each side of the joint being examined (Fig. 10–26). Additional information concerning swelling and tenderness of the proximal interphalangeal joint may be obtained when the examiner places his thumb over the dorsal surface, his index finger over the palmar surface, and the thumb and index finger of his other hand over the medial and lateral aspects of the joint, respectively (Fig. 10–27). Pressure is applied by the digits of the examiner's hands on the dorsal and palmar surfaces to distend the synovial membrane maximally to each side of the joint, where it then may be palpated more easily.

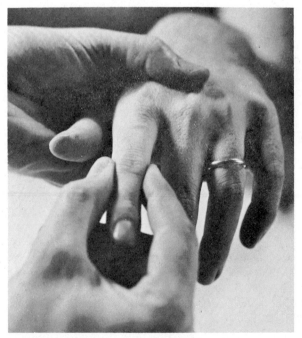

Figure 10–26. Palpation of the proximal interphalangeal joint of the left second finger. The examiner's left hand is supporting the patient's hand while the examiner's right thumb and forefinger are used to palpate simultaneously and alternately the medial and lateral aspects of the joint. The other proximal interphalangeal joints are examined similarly. See text for details.

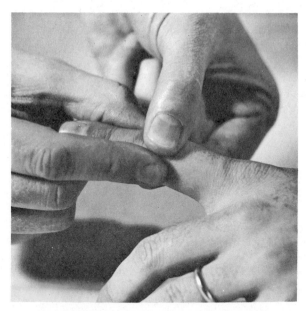

Figure 10–27. An alternate technique for palpation of synovial distention in proximal interphalageal joint is illustrated here on the proximal interphalangeal joint of the second finger on the left hand. The joint capsule is first compressed anteroposteriorly between the examiner's left thumb and second finger while the examiner's right thumb (medial) and second finger (lateral) lightly palpate for fluctuant synovial distention. Then the right thumb and finger compress the joint capsule while the left thumb and finger palpate. The firmness with which pressure is applied in examination of the joint is illustrated by the blanching of the examiner's nails, but for comparison palpation also should be performed gently and lightly.

Distal Interphalangeal Joints

To palpate each distal interphalangeal joint, the examiner places a thumb and index finger on opposite sides of the joint, since articular tenderness, swelling, and local heat are most readily detected on the dorsomedial and dorsolateral aspects of the joint. Hard and usually nontender bony enlargements (Heberden's nodes) are palpated earliest as a ridge over the dorsum of the distal interphalangeal joint but when larger may be more prominently felt medially and laterally. Synovial cysts from joints and tendon sheaths usually have a cystic consistency, which may or may not be compressible and by which they may be recognized; tenderness, local heat, and warmth are usually absent. Synovial cysts of joints develop as an outpouching of the synovial membrane through the articular capsule and are usually located on the dorsal, dorsomedial, or dorsolateral aspect of the joint. Synovial cysts of tendon sheaths usually occur on the palmar or volar aspect of the digit.

Palpation of the nail bed for the presence of clubbing of the fingernails (Fig. 10–12) traditionally has been accomplished using a pulsating depression and release of pressure by the examiner's fingertip on the distal edge of the nail being examined, while another of the examiner's fingertips is placed lightly on the skin fold overlying the nail bed. When clubbing is present, a rocking movement of the nail is transmitted to the proximal edge of the nail bed. To perform this palpation, the examiner holds the nail being examined directly in front of him and both of the examining fingers are pointed toward the patient. This maneuver accurately identifies the location of the proximal edge of the nail. It does not, however, as accurately reveal whether the base of the nail is "floating" in the adjacent loose or edematous soft tissue, which is present when clubbing has occurred. To confirm the presence of clubbing, the examiner palpates the proximal edge of the patient's nail with the tip of one or more fingers or tips of the thumbs pointing distally, as shown in Figure 10–28. When clubbing is definitely present, the proximal nail edge is felt readily and distinctly using this additional technique. Clubbing usually is not painful unless it has developed acutely.

The technique of examining the distal interphalangeal joint is exactly the same as that of examining the proximal interphalangeal joint.

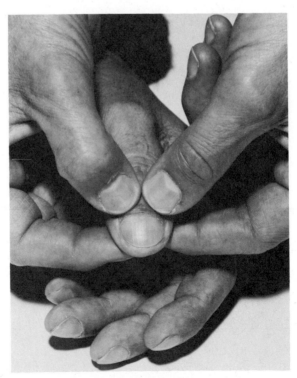

Figure 10–28. Palpation of the proximal edge of the thumbnail for the presence of clubbing. The proximal nail edge can be readily and distinctly felt "floating" in adjacent soft tissue. Note also the clubbing of other fingernails seen in the lower part of the photograph.

However, the examiner should be aware of the marked difference in predilection of the two interphalangeal joints for certain types of disease. Thus, Heberden's nodes and psoriatic arthritis characteristically affect the distal interphalangeal joint, and rheumatoid arthritis commonly involves the proximal interphalangeal joint more than the distal interphalangeal joint. Detachment of the extensor tendon from the base of the distal phalanx produces a flexion deformity of the distal phalanx and hyperextension of the middle interphalangeal joint (mallet finger).

MOVEMENT AND RANGE OF MOTION

Movement of the digits should be evaluated as a unit, and then the movement of each joint can be evaluated separately. A simple measure of over-all function of the fingers is the ability of the patient to make a complete fist and to extend the fingers fully. Movement of the fingers as a whole thus may be observed by asking the patient to flex and then extend his fingers as far as possible (active motion). The thumb should be sufficiently abducted so that it does not interfere with flexion of the fingers or give a misleading impression of a tight fist when the ability to make a fist is actually impaired. A normal, complete fist produced by complete flexion of all the fingers is described as a 100 per cent fist, and a flat hand with no flexion of the fingers would be considered a 0 per cent fist. Examples of approximately 25, 50, and 75 per cent fists are shown in Figure 10–29. Composite flexion of all of the joints of the fingers can also be determined by measuring the distance from the tips of the flexed fingers to the proximal crease of the palm.

The lack of full extension of the fingers is measured best in degrees of full extension that are lacking (for example, the fingers may lack 10, 20, or 30 degrees of full extension). After the patient has flexed and extended his fingers actively, the examiner moves each of the metacarpophalangeal joints to its complete flexion and, while holding the fingers in this position, moves each of the proximal interphalangeal joints to complete flexion and then moves each of the distal interphalangeal joints to complete flexion. The patient's wrist must be extended slightly, and the hand should remain relaxed during these maneuvers in order to evaluate motion of the fingers adequately and correctly. Muscle weakness or "trigger" digits cause limitation of active motion without impairing the range of passive motion. Subluxation of metacarpophalangeal joints is particularly apparent during active flexion of these joints. When this occurs, the distal bone of the metacarpophalangeal joint (proximal end of the adjacent phalanx) should be supported by pressure of the examiner's finger against the palmar aspect of the patient's phalanx throughout the range of passive movement of the metacarpophalangeal joint, in order to reduce the dislocation as much as possible and thereby evaluate more accurately the movement of the joints of the finger distal to the metacarpophalangeal joint.

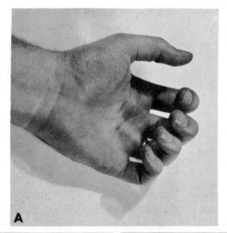

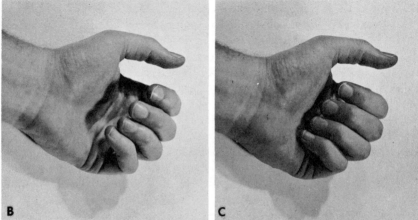

Figure 10–29. Illustrations of approximate degrees of flexion of the fingers used in making a fist. *A.* 25 per cent fist. *B.* 50 per cent fist. *C.* 75 per cent fist. A complete fist (not illustrated) would be recorded as a 100 per cent fist.

Range of Motion

In determining range of motion in individual joints, the examiner should note whether each of the digital joints contributes normally to the total range observed. The proximal interphalangeal joints, for example, may flex completely to enable the fingertips to touch or almost touch the distal portion of the palm, but flexion at the metacarpophalangeal joints may be incomplete. Alternatively, the metacarpophalangeal joints may flex well, but the fingers may be unable to touch the proximal portion of the palm because motion at the proximal interphalangeal joints is limited. Such limitation, however, is not necessarily in the joint.

A greater limitation of passive motion as compared with active motion may occur in any joint affected by pain and swelling. Passive movement of the metacarpophalangeal joints is greater than active movement in the presence of certain types of stenosing tenosynovitis. Rupture of either flexor or extensor tendons also limits active movement of the fingers to a greater degree than it limits passive motion. When the range of motion is limited and voluntary or active motion equals passive motion, the limitation can be attributed to involvement of the joint, to tightening of the articular capsule and periarticular tissues by distention or fibrosis, or to fixed muscle contractures.

The range of motion in the metacarpophalangeal joints results from flexion-extension or abduction-adduction of the proximal phalanges on the metacarpal heads; a combination of these movements allows circumduction. The collateral ligaments are loose in extension and tight in flexion; thus they produce a firm grasp without lateral motion of the fingers when the metacarpophalangeal joint is flexed. The metacarpophalangeal joint of the thumb moves more like a hinge joint, since its lateral motion is restricted. The proximal and distal interphalangeal joints are true hinge joints whose movement is restricted to flexion and extension in contrast to the range of motion in the metacarpophalangeal joints. Hyperextension normally is prevented by the palmar and collateral ligaments. Flexion at the proximal interphalangeal joint is greater than flexion at the distal interphalangeal joint.

To measure the degree of flexion in a joint of any finger, the examiner supports the proximal phalanx while the patient demonstrates range of motion by moving the distal phalanx or phalanges (active motion), or the examiner moves the distal phalanx or phalanges (passive motion). The metacarpophalangeal joints of the fingers flex about 90 degrees from the normal neutral extended position (0 degrees) (Figs. 10–30 and 10–31). The metacarpophalangeal joint of the thumb usually flexes about 50 degrees, but there is more variability in the range of this joint among different people than in the range of the other metacarpophalangeal joints. The proximal interphalangeal joints flex 100 to 120 degrees, and the distal interphalangeal joints flex 45 to 80 degrees from the neutral (0-degree) extended position (Figs. 10–32 and 10–33).

Each metacarpophalangeal joint may hyperextend as much as 30 degrees from the neutral (0-degree) extended position, but some individuals are unable to extend the metacarpophalangeal joint farther than the neutral extended position (Fig. 10–30). The proximal interphalangeal joint rarely hyperextends more than 10 degrees. The distal interphalangeal joint may hyperextend as much as 30 degrees but there is considerable variation, and some individuals cannot extend either joint farther than the neutral extended position. The interphalangeal joint of the thumb commonly hyperextends about 20 to 35 degrees and flexes to about 80 to 90 degrees (Fig. 10–34). Each of the fingers is capable of abduction (spreading of the fingers) and adduction (movement of fingers toward the third or middle finger) when the metacarpophalangeal joint is extended. The complete range of abduction-adduction at the metacar-

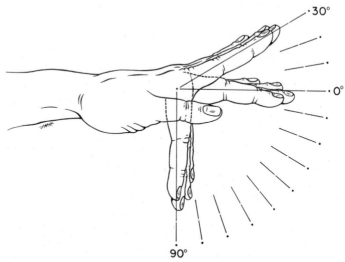

Figure 10–30.   Normal range of flexion and extension in metacarpophalangeal joints of fingers.

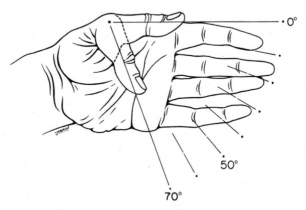

Figure 10–31.   Normal range of flexion in metacarpophalangeal joint in thumb (first digit) usually is about 50 degrees but varies in different people.

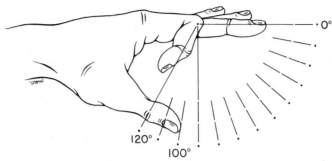

Figure 10–32.   Normal range of flexion in proximal interphalangeal joint.

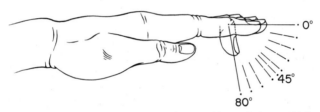

Figure 10–33.   Normal range of flexion in distal interphalangeal joint.

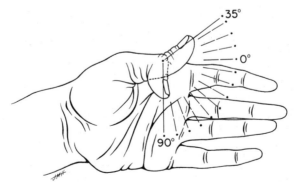

Figure 10–34.   Normal range of flexion and extension in interphalangeal joint of thumb (first digit).

pophalangeal joint is approximately 30 to 40 degrees, but the relative contribution of abduction and adduction varies from joint to joint. There is minimal abduction or adduction at the metacarpophalangeal joint of the thumb, and most of this type of motion in the thumb plus the motion that results from function of the opponens muscle occurs at the carpometacarpal articulation. Abduction at the carpometacarpal articulation may be measured parallel to or at a right angle to the plane of the palm and is about 70 degrees in each plane.

Destruction of the joint and laxity of the articular capsule and ligaments produced by synovial swelling may cause instability of finger joints and eventually lead to dislocation and hypermobile or flail joints. Passive and even active range of motion in a subluxed or dislocated joint can sometimes be tested in the following manner: When the bony structures forming the joint are supported by the examiner in their normal position, the range of motion in the joint may be greater than it is when the joint is subluxed. Considerable improvement in the range of active flexion and extension in a subluxed finger joint when the examiner holds the joint structures in their normal position indicates relatively good potential function of the joint and intact flexor and extensor tendons.

MUSCLE TESTING

A general estimate of the muscular strength of the hands can be made when the patient makes a tight fist by grasping two or more of the examiner's fingers. Another commonly used method of testing grip strength is to have the patient forcefully squeeze a blood pressure cuff that is inflated to 20 mm of mercury. The mean pressure attained by the patient in three attempts can be used in comparative studies. In most patients with diseases involving the muscles or joints, however, the strength of individual muscles of the hands needs to be evaluated separately.

Joints of the Fingers

Flexion of Metacarpophalangeal Joints. The prime movers in flexion of the second through fifth metacarpophalangeal joints are the dorsal interosseous (ulnar nerve, C8) and palmar interosseous (ulnar nerve, C8, T1) muscles. The lumbrical muscles (first and second lumbricals: median nerve, C6, 7; third and fourth lumbricals: ulnar nerve, C8) also flex the metacarpophalangeal joints when the proximal phalangeal joints are in the process of extending. The flexor digitorum superficialis and flexor digitorum profundus muscles are accessory to this motion. Flexion of these metacarpophalangeal joints is tested while the patient sits with his hand and forearm supinated and the forearm resting on a table to

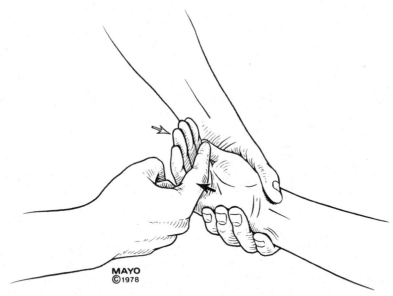

MAYO
©1978

Figure 10–35. Test for flexors of the metacarpophalangeal joints. Patient flexes the fingers while keeping the interphalangeal joints extended. The examiner stabilizes the metacarpals by holding them with one hand and resists flexion with the second (index) finger of the other hand along the proximal row of phalanges.

help stabilize the hand. The patient's metacarpal bones are pressed against the table by the fingertips of one of the examiner's hands or are held between the thumb and fingers of the examiner's hand to stabilize them further. The patient then flexes the metacarpophalangeal joints but keeps the interphalangeal joints extended. Graded resistance against flexion is provided by the examiner's other thumb or fingers placed on the palmar surface of the proximal row of phalanges, as shown in Figure 10–35. Each finger may be tested separately in the same manner if the muscles are of unequal strength.

    Flexion of Proximal Interphalangeal Joints. The prime mover in flexion of the proximal interphalangeal joints of the second through fifth fingers is the flexor digitorum superficialis muscle (median nerve, C7, 8, T1). Flexion of the proximal interphalangeal joints is tested with the patient's hand and forearm supinated and resting on a table with wrist and fingers extended. Each proximal interphalangeal joint should be examined separately. Those not being tested should be held fully extended to minimize the action of the flexor digitorum profundus muscle. The examiner stabilizes the proximal phalanx of the finger being tested by holding it medially and laterally between his thumb and index finger. The patient then flexes the middle phalanx against the graded resistance provided by the fingers of the examiner's other hand, as shown in Figure 10–36.

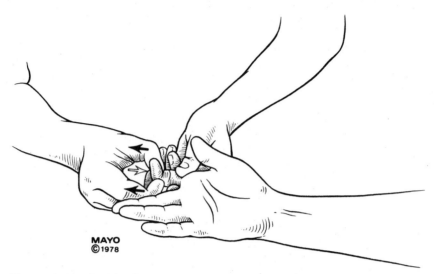

MAYO
©1978

Figure 10–36. Test for flexors of proximal interphalangeal joint. The patient flexes a proximal interphalangeal joint while the examiner stabilizes the proximal phalanx with the thumb and second (index) finger of one hand and provides resistance to flexion with the thumb and finger of the other hand on the sides of the middle phalanx.

Flexion of Distal Interphalangeal Joints. The prime mover in flexion of the distal interphalangeal joints of the second through fifth fingers is the flexor digitorum profundus muscle (second and third fingers: median nerve, C7, 8, T1; fourth and fifth fingers: ulnar nerve, C7, 8, T1). Flexion of the distal interphalangeal joints is tested with the patient's hand supinated and resting as described previously. The examiner stabilizes the middle phalanx of the finger being tested by holding it medially and laterally between his thumb and index finger. The patient then flexes the distal phalanx of the finger against graded resistance provided by the examiner's other hand on the palmar aspect of the patient's fingertip. Each finger should be tested separately.

Extension of Metacarpophalangeal Joints. The prime movers in extension of the metacarpophalangeal joints of the second through fifth fingers are the extensor digitorum communis (radial nerve, C6, 7, 8), the extensor indicis proprius (second finger: radial nerve, C6, 7, 8), and the extensor digiti minimi (fifth finger: radial nerve, C7) muscles. Extension of the metacarpophalangeal joints is tested while the patient's pronated forearm is resting on a table. The patient's hand is held between the thumb and other fingers of the examiner's supinated hand to stabilize the metacarpal bones. The patient's wrist should be slightly extended and the metacarpophalangeal joints flexed. The patient then extends the metacarpophalangeal joints against the graded resistance provided by the fingers of the examiner's other hand pressing on the dorsal surface of the proximal row of phalanges. Each finger should be tested separately.

Extension of Interphalangeal Joints. The prime movers in extension of the proximal and distal interphalangeal joints of the second through fifth fingers are the extensor digitorum communis, extensor indicis proprius, extensor digiti minimi, interosseous and lumbrical muscles. The tendons of the extensor digitorum communis, extensor indicis proprius, and extensor digiti minimi muscles insert on the bases of the middle phalanges and the dorsal digital extensor expansions of the fingers. The dorsal digital expansions are bands of connective tissue and extensor tendons that form a hood over the dorsal surfaces of the metacarpophalangeal joints and digits. They also form the dorsal portions of the capsules of the metacarpophalangeal joints and insert on the bases of the middle and distal phalanges. These muscles are assessed adequately by testing extension of the metacarpophalangeal joints, as described previously.

The interossei originate on the shafts of the metacarpal bones and the lumbricals originate on the flexor digitorum profundus tendons in the palm. Both of these groups of intrinsic hand muscles insert on the dorsal digital extensor expansions of the fingers, and the interossei also insert on the sides of the bases of the proximal phalanges. Thus, the intrinsic muscles simultaneously flex the metacarpophalangeal joints and extend the interphalangeal joints. To test this function of the interossei and lumbricals, the examiner grasps and stabilizes the patient's metacarpal bones with one hand. The patient then actively and simultaneously extends the interphalangeal joints and flexes the metacarpophalangeal joints. The examiner then exerts pressure with the fingers of the other hand, first against the dorsal surface of the patient's middle phalanges in the direction of flexion and second against the palmar surface of the patient's proximal phalanges in the direction of extension. The lumbricals are also evaluated when flexion of the metacarpophalangeal joints is tested, as described in the previous section, and the interossei are evaluated during testing of abduction and adduction of the fingers, as described in the sections that follow.

Abduction. The prime movers in abduction of the second through fifth fingers are the four dorsal interosseous muscles (ulnar nerve, C8, T1) and the abductor digiti minimi muscle (ulnar nerve, C8). Abduction of the fingers is tested while the patient's pronated hand and forearm rest on a table with the fingers adducted. The examiner places the thumb and other fingers of one hand on the patient's metacarpals to stabilize them. The patient then abducts the second through fifth fingers against the graded resistance provided by the examiner's other hand at the sides of the bases of the proximal phalanges, as shown in Figure 10–37. The first and second dorsal interossei are tested by graded manual resistance provided on the radial side of the second and third fingers, respectively. The third and fourth interossei and the abductor digiti minimi muscle are tested by graded manual resistance provided on the ulnar side of the third, fourth, and fifth fingers, respectively.

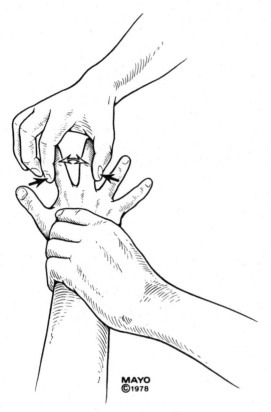

Figure 10–37.   Test for the first and third dorsal interossei. Patient abducts the second (index) and third (middle) fingers while the examiner provides resistance to this movement with the thumb and second finger over the distal portions of the proximal phalanges.

MAYO
©1978

Adduction.   The prime movers in adduction of the fingers are the second, third, and fourth palmar interossei (ulnar nerve, C8, T1). The first palmar interosseous is a small, inconstant muscle involved in movement of the first metacarpophalangeal joint, and it cannot be tested easily. Adduction of the fingers is tested while the patient's pronated hand rests on a table with the fingers in the fully abducted position. The patient is instructed to move the fingers together against the graded resistance provided by the examiner's finger placed at the distal end of a proximal phalanx, as shown in Figure 10–38. Resistance is applied on the ulnar side of the second finger in testing the second palmar interosseous muscle. Resistance is applied on the radial side of the fourth and fifth fingers in testing the third and fourth palmar interossei, respectively. The middle finger has no palmar interosseous muscle and is deviated to either side by the action of the two dorsal interossei that are attached to it, as described in the previous section.

Joints of the Thumb

Flexion of Metacarpophalangeal Joint.   The prime mover in flexion of the metacarpophalangeal joint of the thumb is the flexor pollicis brevis muscle (superficial head: median nerve, C6, 7; deep head: ulnar nerve, C8, T1). The abductor pollicis brevis and adductor pollicis muscles are accessory to this motion. Flexion of the metacarpophalangeal joint of the thumb is tested while the patient's supinated hand and forearm are resting on a table. The distal phalanx should remain relaxed. The examiner holds the first metacarpal between his thumb and index finger to stabilize it and with his other hand provides graded resistance on the palmar surface of the proximal phalanx while the patient flexes the joint.

Flexion of Interphalangeal Joint.   The prime mover in flexion of this joint is the flexor pollicis longus muscle (anterior interosseous branch of the median nerve, C8, T1). Flexion of the interphalangeal joint of the thumb is tested with the patient's supinated hand resting on the table. The examiner holds the proximal phalanx of the thumb to stabilize it. The patient then flexes the distal phalanx in the plane of the palm against graded resistance provided by one finger of the examiner's other hand pressing on the palmar surface of the distal phalanx.

Extension of Metacarpophalangeal Joint.   The prime mover in extension of the metacarpophalangeal joint of the thumb is the extensor

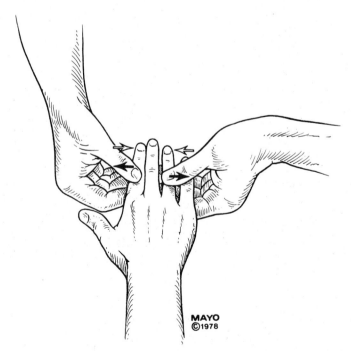

MAYO
©1978

Figure 10-38. Test for the second and third palmar interossei. The patient adducts the second and fourth fingers while the examiner resists this movement with his thumb and fingers at the distal ends of the proximal phalanges of the second (index) and fourth (ring) fingers.

pollicis brevis muscle (radial nerve, C6, 7). The extensor pollicis longus is accessory to this motion. Extension of this joint is tested with the patient's hand resting on its side on the table with the palmar surface perpendicular to the surface of the table. The examiner holds the first metacarpal between one thumb and index finger to stabilize it. The patient then extends the joint in the plane of the palm and away from the table against graded resistance from one finger of the examiner's other hand placed on the dorsal surface of the proximal phalanx.

Extension of Interphalangeal Joint.   The prime mover in extension of the interphalangeal joint of the thumb is the extensor pollicis longus muscle (radial nerve, C6–8). The abductor pollicis brevis and adductor pollicis muscles are accessory to this motion. Extension of this joint is tested with the patient's hand positioned as just described while the examiner holds the sides of the proximal phalanx of the thumb between his thumb and index finger to stabilize it. The patient extends the joint against graded resistance provided by the examiner's fingers placed over the dorsal surface of the tip of the thumb.

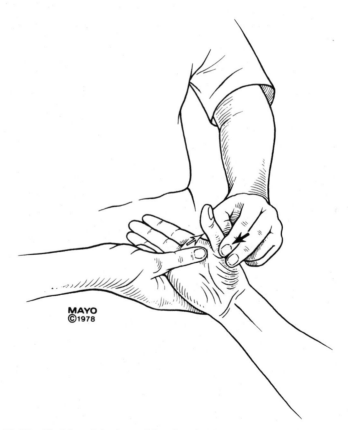

MAYO
©1978

Figure 10–39.   Test for abductors of the thumb. With the hand supinated, the patient abducts the thumb in a vertical plane away from the palm while the examiner provides resistance at the distal end of the first metacarpal.

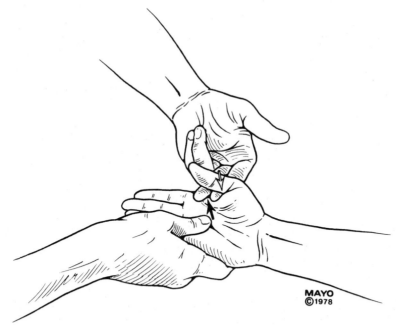

Figure 10–40. Test for adductors of the thumb. With the hand supinated, the patient adducts the thumb in the perpendicular plane toward the palm while the examiner provides resistance to this motion with the fingers of one hand under the proximal phalanx.

Abduction. The prime movers in abduction of the thumb are the abductor pollicis longus (radial nerve, C6, 7) and the abductor pollicis brevis (median nerve, C6, 7) muscles; the palmaris longus muscle is accessory to this motion. Motion takes place primarily at the carpometacarpal joint. Abduction of the thumb is tested with the patient's supinated forearm and hand resting on a table. The patient's wrist is flexed enough to permit the examiner's hand to stabilize the second through fifth metacarpals by grasping them between his thumb and fingers. The patient then raises the thumb in a plane vertical to the palm through the range of abduction. Graded resistance to abduction is provided on the first metacarpal by the fingertips of the examiner's other hand, as shown in Figure 10–39.

Adduction. The prime mover in thumb adduction is the adductor pollicis muscle (ulnar nerve, C8, T1). Motion takes place primarily at the carpometacarpal joint. Adduction of the thumb is tested with the patient's supinated hand resting on a table as described for testing abduction of the thumb. The examiner stabilizes the patient's second through fifth metacarpals by holding them between the thumb and fingers of one hand. The patient then adducts the thumb perpendicularly toward the palm against graded resistance provided at the medial border of the proximal phalanx by one or more fingers of the examiner's other hand (Fig. 10–40). The interphalangeal joint of the thumb should be held in a flexed position to avoid substitution by the extensor pollicis longus.

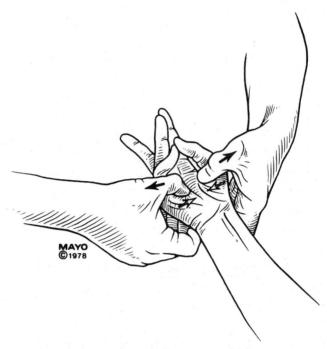

Figure 10–41. Test for opposition of thumb and fifth finger. The patient rotates the palmar surfaces of the distal phalanges of the thumb and fifth finger together while the examiner provides resistance to this motion with the thumbs and fingers of his hands.

Opposition of Thumb and Fifth Finger. The prime movers in opposition of the thumb and fifth finger are the opponens pollicis muscle (median nerve, C6, 7) and the opponens digiti minimi muscle (ulnar nerve, C8, T1); the abductor muscles of the thumb and fifth finger are accessory to this motion. Opposition of the thumb and fifth finger is tested while the patient sits with the supinated hand resting on a table. As the patient brings the palmar surfaces of the distal phalanges of the thumb and fifth finger together, the first and fifth metacarpals rotate toward the midline. The examiner provides graded resistance to this motion by using the thumbs and fingers of his hands placed on the distal ends of the first and fifth metacarpals to rotate and draw the patient's thumb and fifth finger back to their original position, as shown in Figure 10–41. The two opponens muscles are graded separately.

SUGGESTED READING FOR ADDITIONAL INFORMATION

Refer to references at the end of Chapter 9, page 111.

chapter **11**

The Spinal Column

ESSENTIAL ANATOMY

  Vertebrae

  Atlas

  Axis

  Joints of Luschka

  Lumbosacral Articulation

  Sacroiliac Articulation

  Ligaments

  Muscles

  Surface Anatomy

INSPECTION

  Spinal Curvatures

PALPATION AND PERCUSSION

MOVEMENT AND RANGE OF MOTION

  Methods of Determining Range of Motion

    Flexion

    Extension

    Lateral motion

    Rotation

    Cervical motions

    Costovertebral motion

MUSCLE TESTING

SPECIAL EXAMINATIONS OF THE BACK

  Supine Position

    Straight-leg-raising test

    Rocking the pelvis

    Passive extension test

    Hyperextension of an extremity on the vertebral column

  Prone Position

  Side Position

  Sitting Position

ADDITIONAL SPECIAL EXAMINATIONS

  Digital Rectal Examination

  Bimanual Pelvic Examination

  Neurologic Examination

ESSENTIAL ANATOMY

The unique structure of the vertebral column allows flexibility of the trunk and also helps retain an upright posture by means of the coordinated action of muscles, ligaments, and bones. The vertebral column normally has four curves, two with anterior convexities (one in the cervical and one in the lumbar region) and two with posterior convexities (one in the thorax and one in the sacrococcygeal region). The curved shape of the vertebral column and the normally resilient structure of the intervertebral disks help to absorb a substantial degree of shock or concussion. If the curves of the spine are balanced or compensatory as they are in the normal back, the upright position can be maintained with much less muscular effort than when these curves are not balanced or compensated.

Vertebrae

The structure of the vertebrae determines to a great extent the mechanics of the spinal column. A typical vertebra consists of an anterior portion, known as the vertebral body, and a posterior portion, which is the vertebral arch. The vertebral body and adjacent disks are the weight-bearing portions. The size of the vertebral body varies with the weight it supports; it increases in size from the second cervical vertebra to the first portion of the sacrum and then diminishes in size to the tip of the coccyx as the total body weight is transmitted from the lower part of the spinal column to the bony pelvis and lower extremities.

The arches of the vertebrae enclose the spinal cord (Fig. 11–1). Each side of a vertebral arch is formed by a pedicle and a lamina that extends from the pedicle. The laminae from the two sides fuse in the midline posteriorly to complete the posterior boundary of the arch. One bony posterior spinous process and two lateral (or transverse) processes, one on each side, project from the laminae and are the sites of muscle attachments. The spinous process projects dorsally in the midline, where its tip lies subcutaneously and is easily palpable except high in the cervical area. A caudad slant of the spinous process in the thoracic region places the tip of the process at a level opposite the body of the adjacent lower vertebra, but in the lumbar region the spinous process is at a level with the lower portion of its corresponding body. The transverse processes project on each side from the region of the junction of the pedicle and lamina; these are not palpable.

The vertebral arch also supports articular processes that originate from the junctions of the pedicles and laminae. There are four for each vertebra, one projecting downward from each side of the vertebra and one projecting upward on each side of the vertebra to form true or

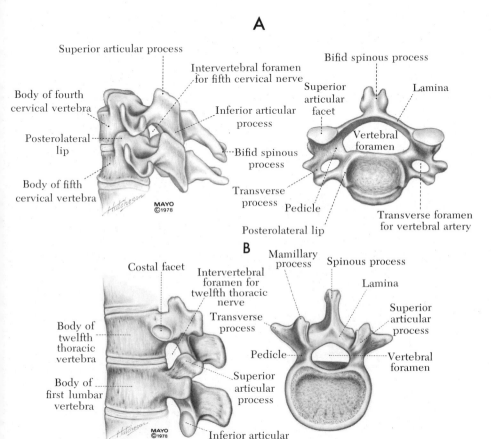

A

Superior articular process

Intervertebral foramen
for fifth cervical nerve

Bifid spinous process

Superior
articular
facet

Lamina

Body of fourth
cervical vertebra

Inferior articular
process

Vertebral
foramen

Posterolateral
lip

Bifid spinous
process

Body of fifth
cervical vertebra

Transverse
process

Pedicle

Transverse foramen
for vertebral artery

Posterolateral lip

MAYO
©1978

B

Mamillary
process

Spinous process

Costal facet

Intervertebral
foramen for
twelfth thoracic
nerve

Lamina

Transverse
process

Superior
articular
process

Body of
twelfth
thoracic
vertebra

Pedicle

Vertebral
foramen

Body of
first lumbar
vertebra

Superior
articular
process

MAYO
©1978

Inferior articular
facet

Figure 11–1. Schematic views of representative vertebrae. *A.* Lateral view of the
fourth (C4) and fifth (C5) cervical vertebrae on the left and the fifth cervical vertebra
from above on the right. The posterolateral lip of C5 articulates with the posterolateral
portion of the inferior aspect of the body of C4. This articulation is known as a joint of
Luschka. *B.* Lateral view of the twelfth thoracic and first lumbar vertebrae on the left
and the first lumbar vertebra from above on the right.

diarthrodial joints between adjacent vertebrae. These joints, known as apophyseal joints and also referred to as articular facets, thus have articular cartilages, thin articular capsules, and synovial membranes. The contact established between the superior articular process of one vertebra with the inferior articular process of the next vertebra above it stabilizes the movement of the vertebrae and particularly prevents forward displacement of a vertebra on the one below it. The angle of the articular surfaces of the apophyseal joints in relation to the horizontal plane of the vertebral bodies varies at different levels and determines to a large degree the type as well as the extent of the movement allowed in various sections of the vertebral column.

The vertebral bodies also articulate with each other by means of a fibrocartilaginous intervertebral disk and thin cartilaginous plates that cover the superior and inferior surfaces of the vertebral body. The cartilaginous plate lies between the disk and the vertebral body. The outer or superficial layers of the intervertebral disk are composed of tough fibers arranged concentrically that form the anulus fibrosus. The center of the disk (the nucleus pulposus) normally is filled with a soft, mucoid substance. The elasticity of the disks permits compression of one edge of the disk and compensatory expansion on the other side of the disk as well as some upward, downward, and rotatory motion between adjacent vertebral bodies. Movement between two adjacent vertebrae is greatest where the disk is thickest, as in the cervical and lumbar regions, and least where the disk is thinnest, as in the thoracic region. The elasticity of the disk provides a cushion or "shock-absorber" effect between adjacent vertebrae, distributes the weight of the body, and thereby prevents concentration of weight on any one edge when the vertebral column is not in an upright position. The disks are thicker ventrally than dorsally in the cervical and lumbar regions and thus contribute to formation of the normal curvature of the spinal column in these areas. Intervertebral disks constitute about one fourth of the total length of the vertebral column above the sacrum.

Atlas

The atlas or first cervical vertebra differs in structure from the other vertebrae in that it lacks a vertebral body and consists only of an anterior and a posterior arch and thickened lateral masses (Fig. 11–2). The atlas is a ring of bone that encloses a central vertebral foramen. The anterior arch forms about one fifth of the circumference of the ring, and the posterior arch forms about two fifths of the circumference; the lateral masses make up the remaining two fifths. The transverse atlantal ligament stretches across the ring of the atlas and divides the vertebral foramen into two unequal parts. The anterior or smaller portion serves as a receptacle for the odontoid process of the axis; the posterior or larger portion encloses the spinal cord. The lateral masses of the atlas rest on

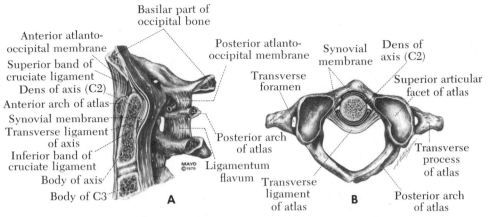

Figure 11–2. *A.* Sagittal section of the first (atlas) and second (axis) cervical vertebrae. *B.* Superior view of the articulation of the atlas and the dens of the axis.

the second cervical vertebra and also support the skull. The skull articulates with the atlas by two joints (the atlanto-occipital joints) formed by the occipital condyles, which project inferiorly on each side from the base of the skull, and the superior articular facets of the atlas, which are directed upward and medially from each lateral mass, forming a cup for the corresponding occipital condyle. These atlanto-occipital joints permit flexion and extension (nodding movements of the head) and slight lateral bending of the head on the neck but very little, if any, rotation of the skull on the atlas, the latter motion being a function of the axis.

Axis

The axis or second cervical vertebra differs from other vertebrae by having a projection from the upper portion of its vertebral body, which is the dens or odontoid process (Fig. 11–2). The axis articulates with the atlas through paired lateral joints and a midline joint formed between the odontoid process and the ring made by the anterior arch and transverse ligament of the atlas. The midline joint (medial atlanto-axial joint) is a trochoid or pivot joint with two synovial cavities, one between the anterior arch of the atlas and the odontoid process and the other between the posterior surface of the odontoid and the transverse atlantal ligament. Each lateral joint also has an articular capsule and synovial membrane. These articulations permit rotation of the skull and atlas on the odontoid process.

Joints of Luschka

The joints of Luschka, also called "lateral intervertebral joints," are very small (only a few millimeters) diarthrodial or, according to some authors, "uncovertebral" joints. They are found only in the cervical portion of the spinal column and correspond to the atlanto-axial and atlanto-occipital articulations rather than to the intervertebral apophyseal articulations. They are located on each side of the cervical intervertebral disks where the lateral borders of the cervical vertebrae project upward to articulate with the beveled inferior lateral portions of the adjacent vertebrae (Fig. 11–1). The joints of Luschka make possible the increased free motion of cervical vertebrae as contrasted with motions of the thoracic and lumbar vertebrae, but as a result of the partial interlocking of adjacent vertebrae provided by the joints of Luschka, the lateral stability of the intervertebral joints of the cervical vertebrae is increased. The joints of Luschka are cupped slightly posteriorly and thus serve as a barrier to posterolateral extrusion of material from the intervertebral disk. Degenerative arthritis with hypertrophic changes and spur formation involving the joints of Luschka is similar to that found in other diarthrodial joints and may cause narrowing of the intervertebral neural foramina with resultant compression of cervical nerve roots.

Some authors have regarded the joints of Luschka as pseudoarthroses or as merely bony protrusions along the lateral edges of the cervical vertebrae that become smooth surfaces through friction and abrasion, rather than as true articulations. Opinions still differ as to whether a synovial lining and articular capsule are present and about the physiology and significance of these structures. In any event, because of their location they are not accessible for physical examination.

Lumbosacral Articulation

The lumbosacral junction is a point of transition between the movable and immovable portions of the spinal column, and its anterior surface is more caudad than its posterior surface. This creates a sharp anteroposterior angulation at the lumbosacral junction that results in the exertion of considerable leverage in this region by the entire length of the vertebral column above the sacrum. A tendency for the fifth lumbar vertebra to sublux anteriorly on the first sacral vertebra as a result of this leverage is countered by the posterior apposition of the articular processes between the fifth lumbar vertebra and the first sacral vertebra. The intervertebral disk at the lumbosacral joint usually is much thicker, especially anteriorly, than other disks and thus provides for extra compressibility as well as greater motion. Besides being particularly vulnerable to the effects of mechanical stresses, the lumbosacral portion of the vertebral column is also a relatively common site of congenital anomalies of the vertebrae and abnormalities of the intervertebral disk.

Sacroiliac Articulation

The sacrum articulates with the bony pelvis of the skeleton by means of a sacroiliac joint on each side of the sacrum. Through these joints the weight of the body above the sacrum is transmitted to the bony pelvis and lower extremities. The upper portion of the sacrum is wider than the lower portion. The sacrum appears to be wedged between the ilia, and its upper end extends farther forward than its lower end.

Each sacroiliac joint is formed by the internal or medial surface of the ilium and the lateral aspect of the first, second, and third sacral vertebrae. The sacroiliac joints have an articular capsule and a synovial membrane. The joint cavity is a narrow, irregular slit, and the articular surfaces of the sacrum and ilium are covered with a layer of cartilage. The lower portion of each sacroiliac joint lies in an anteroposterior plane. The upper portion of the joint is oblique in relation to the frontal plane of the body, and at this level of these joints the ilia are wrapped around the lateral portion of the sacrum posteriorly. The tuberosities of the ilia extend medially beyond the sacroiliac joints and thus cover the upper portions of the joints at the points where the joints are most superficial. A series of strong but short intra-articular fibers (the interosseous sacroiliac ligament) connect the tuberosities of the sacrum and ilium, filling the narrow space between these bones in the posterior portion of the joint. The sacroiliac joints are stabilized by unusually strong, dense, extracapsular ligaments that resist the tendency of the upper end of the sacrum to rotate forward and the lower end of the sacrum to rotate backward during weight-bearing on these joints. Generally, very little motion occurs in these joints; what motion there is disappears with increasing age and usually is gone by middle age.

Ligaments

The vertebrae are bound together by the anterior and posterior longitudinal ligaments, which extend from the sacrum to the base of the occiput. These ligaments greatly increase the stability of the vertebral column. The dense anterior longitudinal ligament is stronger than the posterior longitudinal ligament and limits extension of the vertebral column. The space between the laminae of two adjacent vertebrae is filled by the ligamenta flava, which are thick, paired plates of elastic tissue that help restore the vertebral column to its original postion after bending movements. The spinous processes are connected by the supraspinous and interspinous ligaments, which partially limit flexion and lateral bending of the vertebral column.

Muscles

The large superficial muscles of the back (the trapezius and the latissimus dorsi on each side) almost completely cover the deeper, intrinsic muscles of the back. The latter are composed of an outer layer consisting of the splenius capitis, splenius cervicis, and sacrospinalis muscles on each side and a deeper layer of smaller muscles, including the semispinales, multifidi, rotatores, interspinales, and intertransversarii on each side.

A layer or sheet of lumbodorsal fascia covers the intrinsic muscles of the back and extends upward to the region of the neck, where it becomes continuous with the nuchal fascia. The intrinsic muscles of the back normally function as a unit to control or counteract flexion by extending the vertebral column. The sacrospinalis (also known as the erector spinae) occupies a groove on each side of the spinous processes and extends from the sacrum to the upper cervical vertebrae and base of the skull. These muscles are the longest muscles in the back and are especially well developed and prominent in the lumbar region. Bilateral action of the sacrospinalis muscles counteracts flexion and produces extension or hyperextension of the vertebral column. Muscles attached to the anterior surface of the vertebrae, such as the quadratus lumborum, psoas major, and psoas minor, assist in flexion of the vertebral column. The muscles of the abdominal wall (external oblique, internal oblique, and rectus abdominis) also are important flexors of the spinal column. Abduction (lateral bending) and rotation of the spinal column are performed by contraction of these abdominal and intrinsic back muscles on one side with simultaneous relaxation of the comparable muscles on the opposite side.

Surface Anatomy

Certain easily identified and normally present surface landmarks are useful for orientation in the examination of the back. The spinous processes of the seventh cervical and first thoracic vertebrae are especially prominent in the midline at the base of the back of the neck. The inferior angle of the scapula normally lies at the level of, and lateral to, the interspace between the seventh and eighth thoracic vertebrae. The iliac crest is easily palpable from the posterior to the anterior iliac spines. A line joining the highest point on each iliac crest crosses the body of the fourth lumbar vertebra. The prominences of the spinous processes are usually readily palpable at the bottom of a furrow that runs down the midline of the back from the external occipital protuberance to the middle of the sacrum. On each side of this furrow is a a rounded elevation produced by the sacrospinalis muscle. In the sacral region the furrow becomes shallower, forming a flattened triangular area whose apex lies on the gluteal cleft. The sides of this triangle originate from two symmetric dimples that overlie the posterior superior iliac spines. A line connecting the posterior superior iliac spines crosses the body of the second sacral vertebra. The midportion of each sacroiliac joint lies adjacent and medial to the posterior superior iliac spine on the same side. The upper border of the gluteus maximus muscle arises about 3 cm lateral to the posterior superior iliac spine and runs along the iliac crest; its fibers extend downward and laterally to the prominence of the greater trochanter. A line drawn horizontally at the level of the ischial tuberosities crosses the femurs at the level of the lesser trochanters. The tip of the coccyx lies above the level of the ischial tuberosities.

INSPECTION

Inspection of the back should be made after the patient has removed all clothing, including shoes. The entire back, thighs, legs, hips, and shoulders should be visible. The patient may be draped with a sheet or gown that does not prevent this. When possible, the patient should stand erect with feet together, hips and knees extended, and arms hanging at the sides. The examiner should be far enough away from the patient to permit an initial inspection of the whole back. Some patients need to be allowed a minute or so to assume their natural standing posture before inspection can be evaluated accurately.

Spinal Curvatures

The patient is inspected from behind, from the side, and from the front. From behind, it should be noted whether or not the spine is abnormally curved to one or the other side (scoliosis) or whether there is an exaggeration or flattening of normal anteroposterior curves. Also to be noted are scars, symmetry or asymmetry of the flank, gluteal creases, and iliac crests, differences in the space between the arm and the lateral side of the thorax on the two sides, prominence of one or occasionally of both scapulae, and differences in elevations of the shoulders. When an imaginary vertical line drawn through the sacrum indicates that the prominence of the spinous process of the first thoracic vertebra is not centered over the midline of the sacrum, a listing or tilting of the trunk of the body to one side is present. The degree of listing may be determined by measuring the extent of the deviation of such an imaginary perpendicular line, but the actual degree of deviation may be obscured by compensatory curves. Compensation for scoliosis or lateral curvature of the spinal column is complete when the first thoracic vertebra is centered over the sacrum, regardless of the curvature between these points. Scoliosis is described according to the direction of its convexity. Thus, left lumbar scoliosis would have a convexity of the lumbar curve to the left. Scoliosis may be further defined as functional or structural in type. Functional scoliosis, such as that due to a significant shortening of one leg, will be present when the patient is in the upright position but will disappear when the patient bends forward. This is in contrast to structural scoliosis, which does not disappear in the flexed position and may even be accentuated in this position in comparison with the upright position. Scoliosis in the thoracic region may produce a rotation of the vertebrae that results in a hump or prominence ("gibbus") of the thorax on the side of the convexity. Scoliosis in the lumbar region usually is associated with a prominence of the sacrospinalis muscle on the side of the convexity, but deformity due to a prominence of the vertebrae is less evident in the lumbar region than in the thoracic region. Palpation of the spinous processes is often necessary to confirm the presence or absence of an abnormal spinal curvature suspected from inspection of the back.

A lateral tilt of the pelvis may be observed by comparing the level of the iliac crests when the patient is standing. Normally the superior iliac crests are level, but when the pelvis is tilted laterally, one iliac crest is higher than the other. If the pelvis is tilted to one side, scoliosis is usually present with the convexity facing toward the low side. When a lateral curvature of the spinal column is present and the iliac crests remain level, the deviation of the vertebral column originates within the column itself and cannot be attributed to causes producing a pelvic tilt. When a pelvic tilt and associated scoliosis are caused by a short leg, both can be eliminated by having the patient stand during the examination with a block of wood or other support (such as magazines or books of various thicknesses) under the short leg.

In the forward-bending test, the patient stands facing the seated examiner and then bends forward at the waist keeping his knees straight. The upper extremities are extended loosely in front of the body toward the floor with the fingertips of each hand extended and touching. This position permits the examiner to observe small differences in the rotational dimensions of the thorax. Normally the two sides will be completely symmetric, and deviations from symmetric contours indicate spinal deformity. Scoliosis without rotation is usually postural and much less significant than scoliosis with a rotational abnormality.

Paravertebral muscles in spasm tend to stand out best as delineated muscle masses, which are visible on inspection when the patient is standing and viewed from the back or is in the prone position. The muscles look as though they were being pushed out from beneath the skin on one or both sides of the spinous processes. Paravertebral muscle spasm may be more prominent on one side than the other and is often associated with spasm of the muscles forming the buttock on the involved side (Fig. 11–3). This is relatively common in patients with sciatic pain secondary to a protruded lumbar disk. Asymmetry of the skin folds in the gluteal region may reveal a pelvic tilt or shortness of a lower extremity, as described in Chapter 12.

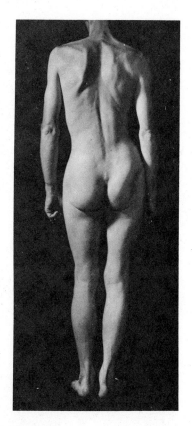

Figure 11–3. Posterior view of the back showing marked paravertebral muscle spasm, which is particularly prominent on the right side and is associated with spasm of the muscles forming the right buttock. A thoracolumbar scoliosis is present with the convexity on the left. The right shoulder is lower than the left. A pelvic tilt is present with the right hip held high. The lateral gluteal skin folds are slightly elevated on the right side. The patient had bilateral sciatica, but it was more marked on the right side and resulted from a midline and right-sided protrusion of the fourth lumbar intervertebral disk.

The presence of subcutaneous fibrous tissue nodules also should be noted. Such nodules are found most often over bony prominences (Fig. 11–4).

When the patient stands and is inspected from the side, the vertebral column has a characteristic thoracic kyphosis (posterior curvature) and a lumbar lordosis (anterior curvature). Any increase or decrease of these curves from normal should be observed. The vertebral column tends to balance anterior and posterior curves; thus, an increase in lumbar lordosis is frequently accompanied by an increase in thoracic kyphosis, and vice versa. Posture may be altered by an increase or decrease in chest development, rounding of the shoulders, protuberance of the abdomen, forward protrusion of the head, and varying degrees of forward tilting of the pelvis (Fig. 11–5). These variations also are noted during inspection from the side.

When kyphosis is present, especially in children, further inspection during the following maneuvers is indicated to determine whether the kyphosis is postural or structural. Correctable postural kyphosis in children can be demonstrated readily by having the child either (1) actively stand straight with abdominal muscles contracted and shoulders pulled back, (2) assume a prone position, or (3) while in the prone position, actively hyperextend the spinal column, lift the head, shoulders, and legs off the examining table to arch the spinal column, and rock on the abdomen. Persistence of kyphosis during these maneuvers indicates a structural or noncorrectable postural kyphosis. Inspection of the patient from the side during forward-bending without bending the knees that reveals a symmetric rounding of the spinal column from shoulders to sacrum without particular accentuation of the bending of any one segment of the spine also indicates a correctable postural type of kyphosis. In contrast, more abrupt bending of a certain segment of the spine may result from compensation for uncorrected structural kyphosis.

In most adults and with advancing age, the thoracic part of the spinal column tends to become more curved, and postural kyphosis may not be correctable because of fixation or limitation of motion that accompanies the aging process. In such patients kyphosis is usually mild and often familial.

Observation of the patient from the front for evidence of abnormalities associated with involvement of the spinal column completes the inspection of the spine. If the patient is draped with a sheet or gown, the drape should be removed or drawn to the midline to permit adequate

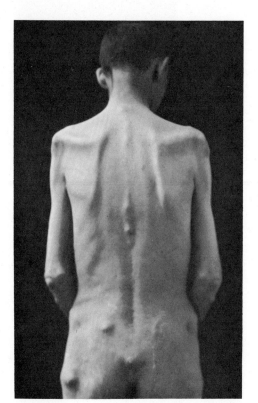

Figure 11-4. Multiple subcutaneous rheumatoid nodules over bony prominences on back, pelvis, and hips of a patient with chronic, debilitating rheumatoid arthritis.

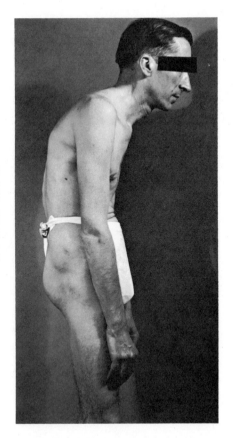

Figure 11-5. Lateral view of patient with ankylosing spondylitis showing forward protrusion of head, flattening of anterior chest wall, thoracic kyphosis, protrusion of abdomen, fixed abdominal creases resulting from kyphosis, and flattening of lumbar lordosis. This patient also has slight flexion of the hips on the pelvis.

inspection of spinal abnormalities. Nutritional status, general body type, symmetry or asymmetry of trunk and extremities, postion of the head and neck, and the level of the nipples and shoulder are sometimes more evident in this view, but actual structural abnormalities of the spinal column are best determined from the lateral or posterior views. The patient's gait and walking posture should be observed from the front, side, and back. Inspection also should include observation of the manner in which the patient sits and moves from sitting to standing to lying down and arising again. Inspection of irregularity of motion in the upper cervical portion of the spinal column in atlanto-axial subluxation is described on page 178, along with other special tests of cervical vertebrae.

PALPATION AND PERCUSSION

Palpation and percussion of the back may produce pain or reveal tenderness of abnormal structures. However, since abnormalities of different structures in the back may produce similar symptoms, it is important that the examiner evaluate these structures in a systematic fashion and recheck positive findings to confirm initial impressions. Pain or tenderness during palpation or percussion of the back may originate as follows:

1. Abnormalities of joints and adjacent bones may produce pain or localized tenderness. For example, low back pain may result from involvement of the sacroiliac joints, degenerative changes in the lumbar vertebrae, or a localized destructive process in a vertebra or intervertebral disk.

2. Muscle spasm in the region of the back is a common source of pain and may make evaluation of underlying structures by palpation or percussion difficult or even impossible. Muscle spasm may result from degenerative or inflammatory processes in muscle fibers or, secondarily, from misuse of muscles resulting in sustained contractions. It also is seen often in chronic or acute anxiety states. Secondary muscle spasm may accompany painful lesions in structures adjacent to involved muscles and sometimes produces tenderness along the sites of muscle attachments to bones.

3. Referred nerve pain, which often is transient and shooting but may be persistent, characteristically occurs along the distribution of a particular nerve root. An example is sciatic nerve pain that accompanies a protruded intervertebral disk in the lumbar region. This type of pain occurs even when adjacent muscles are as relaxed as they can be. Referred pain to the back from abdominal visceral diseases usually produces pain and muscle spasm localized to one spot in the distribution of the affected nerve arc.

4. Low back pain also may result from tenderness of localized soft-tissue structures, such as fat pads, ligaments, and tissues overlying bony structures such as spinous processes.

Palpation

Back. Palpation of the back while the patient is standing, lying prone, and sitting provides information that supplements the findings from palpation in any one position. When a patient is tense or muscle spasm is present, palpation while the patient is prone is more satisfactory than if he is in any other position. A pillow under the abdomen to support the spinal column is desirable; the pillow not only flattens the lumbar lordosis but also separates the spinous processes so that they can be identified more easily.

The patient is directed to point out areas of tenderness or discomfort as specifically as possible before the examination is started. The diffuseness or specificity of such subjective localization can be of considerable significance when correlated with the physical findings. Palpation of the back is performed gently with the examiner's fingertips and thumbs slightly bent and probing through layers of skin, subcutaneous tissues, muscles (including their insertions), and bony prominences while the patient is as relaxed as possible. During palpation, the findings are noted in reference to the anatomic landmarks of the back described previously. Palpation of subcutaneous tissues in an area removed from the patient's localization of discomfort helps to accustom the patient to the examination and enables the examiner to evaluate the patient's pain threshold and general demeanor and reactivity as well as the tone of muscles and the subcutaneous turgor. Areas of localized tenderness not previously described by the patient may be found, and the presence of any local heat, nodules, fat pads, or masses should be noted. When fat tissue or tight muscles offer extra or excessive resistance, the fingers of one of the examiner's hands may be placed on top of the other hand to utilize their combined pressure.

In general, palpation is performed from the top downward or vice versa and from side to side at various levels. The posterior aspect of the vertebral column is palpated for evidence of abnormal prominence of any spinous process; this may indicate a collapsed vertebral body from mechanical, metabolic, infectious, inflammatory, or malignant disease. A bony shelf or abnormal projection of one vertebra in relation to its adjacent vertebrae suggests subluxation or spondylolisthesis. The usual sites of spondylolisthesis are the fifth lumbar vertebra, which is displaced forward over the body of the sacrum, and the fourth lumbar vertebra, displaced forward over the fifth. Any other bony irregularities should be palpated; these are especially prominent at the lumbosacral level and in the regions of the spinous processes, scapulae, and shoulder girdle. When palpation over the attachments of the gluteal muscle and the lumbosacral joints reveals muscles in spasm, the muscles are likely to be tender and feel abnormally tight and contracted. Muscles such as the sternocleidomastoid and the upper trapezius and skin folds may be examined by gripping them between the thumb and second finger; this is done best when the patient is supine or prone.

Excessive muscle spasm produces pain and tenderness in the distribution of the involved muscle. In such instances the original site of pain often cannot be determined accurately until the muscle has been relaxed. Thus it may be necessary to re-examine the patient after a period of rest in bed when a more comfortable position can be attained. When excessive spasm exists, it is best to defer conclusive evaluation of the spinal examination until it can be performed more reliably.

Gluteal Muscle Attachments. Tenderness of the gluteal muscle attachments also can be evaluated best with the patient lying on his abdomen. Palpation is carried out with the leg in active hyperextension. The patient is directed to raise his leg (with the knee extended) high enough off the table to cause contraction and tightening of the gluteal muscles in order to exert a pull on muscle attachments, but the leg should not be raised high enough to mobilize the pelvis or lumbar vertebrae, since disorders of these structures may produce symptoms and thus prevent localization of pain. If the gluteal muscle attachments are involved, this maneuver should reproduce the patient's pain, and localized palpation over the superior attachments of the gluteal muscles will help differentiate this pain from other sites of subcutaneous tenderness.

Fat Pads and Adipose Tissue. These may be the sites of localized tenderness, especially in the gluteal muscle and lumbosacral regions. The tenderness may be localized or may involve adipose tissues more diffusely. Fat pads or adipose tissue can be evaluated best by grasping these tissues between the examiner's finger and thumb and palpating them specifically for tenderness. The examiner can evaluate tender areas further by moving the skin and superficial fatty tissues to one side with one hand while palpating underlying structures with the other hand. If the underlying structures are not tender, the tenderness that has been demonstrated previously must involve the superficial tissues that were moved aside by the examiner.

Palpation for atlanto-axial subluxation is described on page 178 with other special tests of the cervical vertebrae.

Percussion

Percussion is performed with the patient standing or sitting. In either instance the patient should be leaning slightly forward to make percussion of spinous processes and the spaces between them easier and more precise. It may be helpful to compare these results with the findings obtained from percussion with the patient in a prone position. A small pad under the abdomen of a prone patient will accomplish the desired separation of the spinous processes.

Percussion is performed manually or with a percussion hammer over the vertebrae and spinous processes in both painless and painful areas to appraise the patient's tolerance of discomfort. Examination by percussion should include the lumbosacral joint, sacroiliac joints, spinous processes, and the sacral attachments of the latissimus dorsi. As with palpation, this can be done from the top downward or vice versa and from side to side, but in any event percussion should be performed systematically to avoid omission of any particular area.

Mild jarring of the spinous processes with the ulnar aspect of the examiner's fist may reveal generalized or localized tenderness but does not distinguish between the pain of muscle spasm and the pain of intrinsic disease or abnormality of bony structures. When generalized tenderness is found by this means, more accurate localization should be attempted by careful percussion of the region with the tip of the examiner's third (middle) finger. If the examiner's third (middle) finger is placed over a spinous process and is percussed while the second and fourth fingers of the same hand are placed on either side of the spine, paravertebral muscle spasm may be readily detected and localized by the reaction felt by the second and fourth fingers. Pain that is accompanied by muscle spasm prevents accurate localization, but localized pain in the absence of muscle spasm often represents a significant abnormality of the structures in the area being examined. The use of the three fingers spaced apart as described also permits more accurate localization of painful areas detected by percussion.

Jarring of the spinal column can be accomplished also by having the standing patient rise to his toes and then forcibly drop back to the floor on his heels. This type of percussion maneuver may indicate in general whether pain or tenderness is present in the spinal region and occasionally helps in the localization of pain; however, more specific localized percussion as described usually is required.

MOVEMENT AND RANGE OF MOTION

The vertebral column permits extension (bending backward), flexion (bending forward), abduction (bending to either side), and rotation. The extent of these movements varies in different regions of the vertebral column. Movement of the spinal column is greatest in the cervical region, is more restricted in the lumbar and thoracic regions, and is not present in the sacral region. Mobility in the vertebral column depends primarily on the thickness and elasticity of the intervertebral disks, the position and direction of the interarticular facets, and the limitations established by the vertebral ligaments. Age, sex, general physical condition, and previous or unusual physical activity are also significant factors that affect spinal movement. Spinal mobility varies considerably among normal individuals and among different racial groups. Movement of the vertebral column as a whole should be differentiated from movement that takes place primarily in certain segments such as the cervical or lumbar regions. Forward bending usually includes both flexion of the hips and of the vertebral column, and it is difficult to separate the two components without fixation of the pelvis by the examiner in order to assess just the range of spinal flexion. The values used to assess the range of spinal motion generally are only approximations for adults up to middle age. There is a tendency for spinal mobility to decrease after middle age.

Flexion occurs primarily in the cervical, low thoracic, and lumbar regions. Flexion of the vertebral column as a whole produces the greatest range of motion. From the neutral or upright position, the column as a whole usually flexes to about 90 degrees. If the cervical portion is not included in the movement and the pelvis is stabilized, the trunk flexes about 40 degrees.

Extension of the vertebral column takes place mainly in the cervical and lumbar regions. If the cervical portion is not included in the measurement, the trunk extends about 30 degrees from the neutral or upright position.

In order to maintain balance, the pelvis normally shifts in the opposite direction as the trunk moves backward or forward.

The vertebral column as a whole bends about 50 degrees to either side; this occurs mostly in the cervical, low thoracic, and lumbar regions. If cervical motion is excluded, lateral motion of the low thoracic and lumbar portions is about 30 to 40 degrees to each side.

Rotation is most marked in the cervical region and is relatively restricted in the lumbar and thoracic regions. If motion of the neck is excluded and the pelvis is stabilized, the vertebral column rotates about 30 degrees to each side.

Methods of Determining Range of Motion

Spinal motion is determined from the positions used for inspection. When the examiner is seated behind the standing patient, he can stabilize the patient's extremities by adducting his own knees and legs against the patient's legs and thus can detect or prevent any movement of the patient's legs during examination of motion of the vertebral column. Spinal bending should be performed without permitting the patient to bend his knees or hips. When the examiner is standing behind or alongside the patient, he can stabilize the patient's hips and pelvis by holding the pelvis firmly with his hands and arms in a hugging type of grasp while the patient bends forward.

Flexion. When bending forward, the patient should flex his head and neck as well as the other segments of the vertebral column and let his arms hang at the sides of his body or fall forward with the bending motion. With the motion of this maneuver the lumbar lordotic curve normally will first flatten and then flex slightly, as the amount of forward bending increases. Normally, the flexed position when viewed from the side forms a smooth curve extending from the sacrum to the base of the skull (Fig. 11–6). A persistent flattening or lordosis of the lumbar region while the patient is bending forward indicates an abnormal loss of motion in this portion of the spinal column. Whether this abnormality is intrinsic or results from muscle spasm can often be best evaluated by viewing the spinal column from the side. Abnormal prominences or sharp angulations of the vertebral column also may be detected from a side view.

Normal spinal flexion is a straightforward motion. Lateral or rotatory deviations during flexion usually indicate asymmetric muscle spasm but do not indicate the reason for the spasm.

Movement of the spinal column also may be evaluated by palpation of the separation of the lumbar spinous processes, which normally occurs during flexion. This is accomplished when the examiner places two or more fingers of one hand on adjacent spinous processes and observes the range of spread of the fingers during spinal flexion. Failure of the spinous processes to separate indicates limitation of motion.

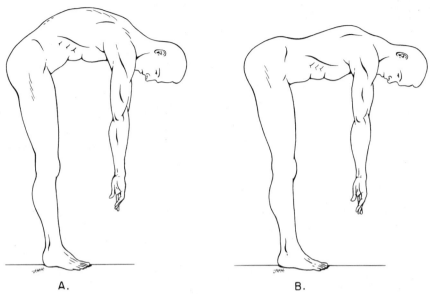

A.   B.

Figure 11-6. Forward bending positions. *A.* Normally on bending forward the entire spinal column has a smooth curved contour when viewed from the side. *B.* A persistence of the lumbar lordotic curve while bending forward indicates limitation of functional motion in the lumbar vertebrae. Note that the motion of flexion is all taking place in the hip joints. This abnormality is characteristic of conditions associated with marked spasm of paravertebral muscles.

The degree of spinal flexion plus flexion of the hips is often recorded by measuring the distance from the fingertips to the floor, specifying the number of centimeters ahead of the toes that is used for the site of the measurement. However, if only the range of spinal motion is being determined, this is not accurate, because the floor-touching test gauges flexibility but does not consider differences of height or structure. Various graphic devices or arbitrary grading systems also can be used to record range of spinal motion, but careful measurement of height without shoes is a satisfactorily accurate method of determining changes in spinal curves or motions in an individual patient over a period of time.

Extension. The degree of extension of the vertbral column is determined by having the patient bend backward. During this motion, the patient stands with both feet on the floor, and the examining physician stabilizes the pelvis by firm pressure with his fist against the patient's sacrum and by counterpressure with his other hand on the upper anterior portion of one of the patient's thighs. Normally the trunk will extend about 30 degrees from the upright position (Fig. 11–7). Extension usually increases the lordotic lumbar curve, straightens out the thoracic part of the vertebral column, and tilts the head backward. Failure to increase the lordotic lumbar curve indicates limitation of motion in this portion of the spinal column. The degree of spinal extension can be measured by various graphic devices,

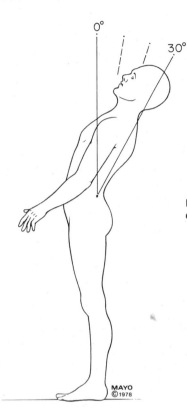

Figure 11-7. Schematic drawing of normal extension of the vertebral column.

or spinal motion can be estimated by percentages of normalcy or arbitrary grades.

Lateral Motion. Lateral motion of the spinal column is determined when the patient bends to one side and then to the other (Fig. 11-8). At times the pelvis may be stabilized more satisfactorily for lateral bending if the feet are separated 50 to 60 cm than if they are together. The normal spinal column has a smooth, lateral curve of about 50 degrees from the upright position extending from the sacrum to the base of the skull (Fig. 11-8). Sharp angulations, pain, and muscle spasm during lateral spinal motion as well as during flexion and extension are abnormal and should be noted. Normally the degree of lateral motion is equal on both sides; inequality of motion indicates functional restriction of motion on one side. When the arc of the curve of the spinal column is greater while the patient is bending to one side than it is while he is bending to the other, abnormal movement is also indicated.

Rotation. Rotation is evaluated when the patient rotates the trunk to one side and then to the other while his legs and pelvis are stabilized by the examiner's manual restraint (as described previously) while the patient remains in a standing position or by having the patient sit with arms and forearms crossed over each other across the anterior wall of the chest. Rotation takes place primarily in the thoracic and cervical regions. The trunk can rotate about 90 degrees to either side; however, if neck motion is excluded and the pelvis is stabilized, the low thoracic and lumbar portions rotate only about 30 degrees to either side. Loss of rotation suggests involvement primarily of the thoracic portion of the spinal column in conditions such as ankylosing spondylitis, for example.

Cervical Motions. Cervical motions are evaluated in either the standing or the sitting position. The patient tips his head forward for flexion, backward for extension, and for rotation turns his head to each side as if looking over each shoulder. Lateral motion is determined when the patient tries to touch his ear to his shoulder without raising the shoulder girdle. Normally the cervical portion of the spine allows about 45 degrees of flexion, 50 to 60 degrees of extension, 60 to 80 degrees of rotation, and 40 degrees of lateral bending. The atlanto-occipital joint permits most of the motions of flexion and extension, and the atlanto-axial joint permits rotation. Lateral motion of the neck occurs primarily below the atlas from the

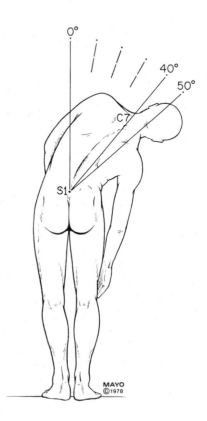

Figure 11–8. Schematic drawing showing normal lateral motion of spine (measured from a mark identifying the first sacral vertebral prominence, S1).

motions of the second to seventh cervical vertebrae. Thus, the specific limitation of motion observed in the neck indicates the part of the cervical spinal column involved.

The location of neck pain that occurs during lateral cervical motion may be of considerable help in differentiating the pain of muscle spasm from that due to involvement of the spinal apophyseal joints. When pain is felt on the side toward which the neck is tilted, involvement of the apophyseal joints is suggested, since this motion compresses the articular facets on the same side, thereby aggravating any already existing irritation of the nerve roots. By contrast, when neck pain occurs on the side opposite the one toward which the neck is rotated, muscle or ligamentous pain is suggested, since the muscles and ligaments on that side of the neck are stretched by this motion.

Forward protrusion of the head, observable on inspection (p. 161), or the range of cervical flexion and extension can be measured by recording the distance between the occiput and a wall when the patient is standing with his back to the wall and with both heels as close as possible to the junction of the wall and the floor. The patient then is instructed to extend his neck without raising his chin beyond a horizontal level in order to bring his head as close as possible to the wall.

Costovertebral Motion. Costovertebral motion is determined by measuring chest expansion during inspiration and expiration. This may be estimated by inspection of the patient during deep inspiration and expiration from the back and sides while the examiner's hands are placed on either side of the lower posterolateral portion of the thorax; expansion of the chest thus can be both seen and felt. However, measurement of chest expansion with a nonelastic tape measure is easy and is a more accurate method of measurement. Different absolute measurements of chest expansion will be found at various levels of the thorax and may account for differences noted by different examiners if this factor is not considered. The nipple line in males or just above it in females is a generally satisfactory and recommended standard site for measurement of chest expansion. The degree of chest expansion, like other spinal motions, varies with age and general physical condition, but normally it is at least 5 to 6 cm in young adults and may be up to 10 to 13 cm in some individuals.

Various instruments, such as those designated as "spondylometer," "inclinometer," and "tiltometer," have been devised in an attempt to standardize measurements of spinal motion and posture, especially for serial examinations. Grid graph photographs, measurements using skin markers, plumb line strings, or tapes, and formulae to calculate and evaluate spinal angles have also been proposed. All have some advantages as well as disadvantages, but their usefulness is often limited to certain diseases and disorders. No one method appears as yet to have achieved widespread acceptance or use or to have supplanted the careful, experienced performance of physical examination techniques.

MUSCLE TESTING

Flexion of the Neck.   The prime movers in flexion of the neck are the sternocleidomastoid muscles (accessory nerve, spinal part, C2, 3). The longus capitis, longus colli, scalenus group, infrahyoid group, and rectus capitis anterior are accessory muscles. Flexion of the neck is tested with the patient supine. The examiner places one hand on the lower midthorax to stabilize it. The patient then flexes the neck through the range of motion against graded resistance provided by the examiner's other hand on the forehead. By flexing the neck with the head rotated to one side, the sternocleidomastoid muscle on the side away from the rotated head may be tested separately, as shown in Figure 11–9.

Extension of the Neck.   The prime movers in extension of the neck are the superior fibers of the trapezius (accessory nerve, spinal part, C3, 4), semispinalis capitis (dorsal rami of spinal nerves), splenius capitis (dorsal rami of the middle and lower cervical nerves), erector spinae (adjacent spinal nerves), and semispinalis cervicis (dorsal rami of spinal nerves)

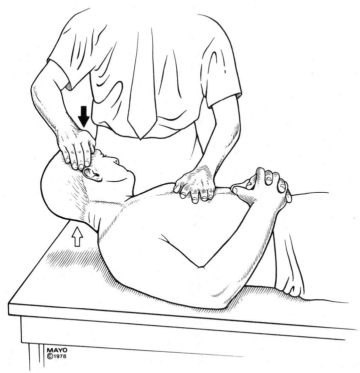

Figure 11–9.   Test for the right sternocleidomastoid muscle. The patient rotates the head to the left and flexes the neck to raise the head from the table. Resistance to this motion is provided to the examiner's hand on the side of the patient's head. The left sternocleidomastoid muscle can be tested when the patient's head is rotated to the right.

muscles. Extension of the neck is tested with the patient prone. The examiner places one hand high on the midthorax (in the region of the scapulae) to stabilize it. The patient then extends the cervical spine through the range of motion while the examiner provides graded resistance against the occiput with his other hand.

Flexion of the Trunk. The prime mover in flexion of the trunk is the rectus abdominis muscle (ventral rami of thoracic nerves, T6–12). The internal and external oblique muscles of the abdomen are accessory to this motion. Flexion of the trunk is tested with the patient in the supine position with hands clasped together behind the head. The examiner stabilizes the lower part of the body by holding the legs firmly, and the patient flexes the thorax on the pelvis through the range of motion by moving up toward the sitting position. Flexion of the trunk can be considered normal if the patient is able to rise to a sitting position while keeping the vertebral column flexed.

Rotation of the Trunk. The prime movers in rotation of the trunk are the external and internal oblique muscles of the abdomen (ventral rami of thoracic nerves, T8–12; iliohypogastric nerve, T12, L1; ilioinguinal nerve, T12, L1). The latissimus dorsi, multifidus, rotator, semispinalis, and rectus abdominis muscles are accessory to this motion. Rotation of the trunk is tested with the patient in the supine position with hands clasped together behind the head. The examiner stabilizes the legs by holding them firmly, as described for flexion, and the patient rotates and flexes the thorax first to one side and then to the opposite side. To test the right external oblique and left internal oblique muscles, the patient rotates and flexes the thoracolumbar spine toward the left, as shown in Figure 11–10. To test the left external oblique and right internal oblique muscles, the patient rotates and flexes the thoracolumbar spine toward the right. Rotation can be considered normal if the patient is able to rotate and elevate the upper part of the trunk off the table and hold the position shown in Figure 11–10.

Extension of the Trunk. The prime movers in trunk extension are the erector spinae (adjacent spinal nerves) and quadratus lumborum (lumbar plexus, T12, L1, 2) muscles. Extension of the trunk is tested with the patient in a prone position with arms at the sides. The examiner immobilizes the pelvis by pressing down firmly with one hand and forearm across the upper parts of the thighs or buttocks. The patient then extends the thoracolumbar spine by raising the thorax off the table against graded resistance provided by the examiner's other hand over the midthorax in the scapular region.

SPECIAL EXAMINATIONS OF THE BACK

Many types of special examinations of the vertebral column have been described. Although one or more of these special tests may aid in establishing the correct diagnosis, single special tests are usually not specific

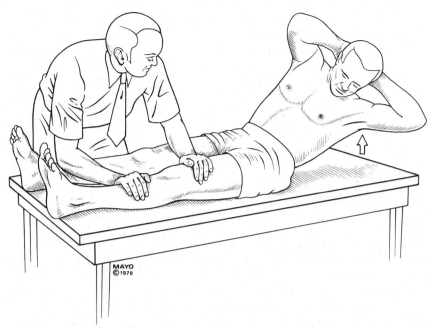

Figure 11–10. Test for rotators of the trunk. In the supine position, the patient flexes and rotates the trunk to the left and holds the position shown to demonstrate normal strength of the right external oblique and left internal oblique muscles.

enough to be diagnostic or completely reliable in establishing either the site or nature of the lesion. Likewise a single test, especially if it is negative, often does not exclude the particular condition for which the test has been proposed.

Certain special tests discussed next are grouped according to the position of the patient while they are performed. Many of these tests have eponymic synonyms. These are omitted wherever possible, because the eponym is less descriptive and sometimes confusing.

Supine Position

Straight-Leg-Raising Test. This test is carried out by the examiner while the patient's leg and thigh are as relaxed as possible. The examiner places one hand under the patient's heel and holds the foot firmly in dorsiflexion by exerting pressure cephalad from this grasp. While the examiner gradually and passively flexes the thigh on the pelvis by moving the foot, the examiner's other hand is placed just above the patella of the side being tested, and with it he exerts gentle but firm downward pressure to hold the knee fully extended. The limit of the angle of flexion is measured by the degrees in the angle formed between the surface on which the patient is lying and the elevated lower extremity. The patient's other leg and thigh should be stabilized in extension while this test is being performed. The angle at which pain, muscle spasm, or flexion of the pelvis occurs is compared with that observed on similar examination of the opposite lower extremity.

Elevation of the lower extremity produces tension on the sciatic nerve and hamstring muscles, but normally each leg and thigh can be raised almost to a right angle without discomfort. When this examination causes pain in the region of the hip or low in the back and limitation of flexion at the hip in the extremity being examined, the test is considered "positive" and suggests nerve root irritation or muscle spasm on the painful side. When dorsiflexion of the foot of the extremity being tested increases the discomfort of the straight-leg raising test, this discomfort is thought to be a further indication of nerve root irritation; no increase in pain suggests a discomfort of muscular origin. Straight-leg-raising flattens the lumbar part of the vertebral column, stretches the ligaments and extensor muscles of the hip and thigh, and when painful may suggest an abnormality of the lumbo-sacral or sacroiliac regions rather than of the sciatic nerve. Occasionally, the straight-leg-raising test will produce pain in the sacral, gluteal, or posterior thigh regions on the side opposite to the one being examined. This also suggests nerve root irritation on the painful side. When this occurs, straight raising of the other leg also will cause pain in the same area. Mild discomfort behind the knee may be described by the patient as due to tightening of the hamstrings or disease of the knee or popliteal area, but this should not be considered a positive response to the test.

When restriction of motion is observed, it is helpful for the examiner to perform the straight-leg-raising test slowly with one hand and to palpate muscle spasm and movement of the spinal column with his other hand, which is placed under the patient's lower vertebrae. If pain and muscle spasm occur low in the back before spinal movement is detected, a sacroiliac lesion is suggested. Pain after motion of the lumbar vertebrae is consistent with either lumbosacral or sacroiliac involvement.

Rocking the Pelvis.   A form of passive movement of the lower part of the spinal column can be tested as follows: The examiner or the patient partially flexes the patient's knees; then the examiner places one arm under both thighs. The patient's thighs and lower part of the spinal column are flexed maximally, bringing both knees as close to the abdomen as possible. With the patient's legs in this position, the patient's pelvis is moved from side to side and also rotated back and forth on the spinal column by the examiner. Normally this rocking motion of the pelvis is painless. Thus, the presence and location of pain resulting from either lateral or rotatory motions may be helpful in detecting and localizing significant involvement of the lumbar and lumbosacral portions of the spinal column. This maneuver also may produce or accentuate sciatic pain and hence should always be performed with caution.

Passive Extension Test.   To perform this test, the patient is moved to one end of the examining table so that the pelvis is at the edge of the table and the legs can be dropped down over the end of the table. When the leg on the involved side is lowered, pain develops in the sacral, gluteal, or posterior thigh region and is relieved by flexion of the unaffected leg while the affected leg is still down. Many lesions of the back or fascial contractures of the anterior portion of the thigh may cause some localized pain with this maneuver, but the procedure is of most significance when sciatic pain is present and sciatic radiation of pain results from the maneuver.

Hyperextension of an Extremity on the Vertebral Column. To test more specifically for abnormality of the *sacroiliac joints,* the patient is moved to one side of the examining table so that he lies with one leg and buttock close enough to this edge that the extremity can be let down over the side of the table to produce hyperextension of this extremity on the vertebral column. During this test the patient's pelvis and lumbar spine are held in a fixed position by having the patient grasp the other lower extremity just below the knee and with clasped hands flex the hip so that the thigh lies as much as possible against the abdomen. The examiner assists in this fixation of the patient's pelvis and lumbar vertebrae by placing one hand over the patient's clasped hands after the hip joint has been flexed. With the other hand the examiner then lowers the patient's leg on the side being examined so that both the leg and the thigh project over the edge of the table and gradually hyperextend the hip joint as far as possible.

The procedure is repeated for the other extremity by having the patient move across the examining table so that the opposite extremity can be let down over the side of the table after fixation of the spinal column and pelvis, as just described. If the sacroiliac joint is the site of pain, this maneuver accentuates the pain in the region of the sacroiliac joint on the side of the hyperextended thigh. The test may be positive for unilateral or bilateral involvement of the sacroiliac joints.

Prone Position

Hyperextension of Back. This test should be performed with the patient's arms in adduction and at the sides of his body with the palms of the hands next to the thighs in the resting position. The patient is instructed to raise his head, shoulders, and arms from the examining table as in arching or hyperextending the spinal column. The examiner stabilizes the patient's legs by exerting downward pressure with his hands on the thighs during this maneuver. The patient then relaxes and, after assuming the resting position again, is instructed to keep one leg extended while actively hyperextending each leg in sequence. These procedures may help the patient and the examiner to localize painful areas in the back to either bone or muscle. When the localization is referable to muscles, the pain produced by active hyperextension of the back by this maneuver is primarily in the attachment of the latissimus dorsi muscle, whereas the pain resulting from active hyperextension of the leg as described is primarily in attachments of the gluteus maximus muscles. It is advisable not to perform hyperextension of the back vigorously unless x-ray examination of this region has been obtained, since this maneuver may aggravate intrinsic bony lesions.

A procedure for evaluating tenderness of the gluteal muscle attachments also was described in the section on palpation of the back. It should be mentioned that active hyperextension of the leg in the prone position also is painful when the *psoas muscle* is abnormal on the side of the elevated leg.

Useful information concerning *painful muscle spasm* in the back can be obtained sometimes when the examiner raises both of the patient's legs off the table by placing one arm under the legs at the level of the knees (or just above the knees if necessary for adequate leverage) and palpates the lower portion of the back and spinal column with his other hand. If the patient pushes down on the examiner's arm that is being used to elevate the lower extremities by attempting to flex his hips, more complete relaxation of paravertebral and gluteal muscles may be obtained. This maneuver shortens the intrinsic muscles of the back and helps relieve muscle tension and spasm; it permits more accurate localization of tenderness by palpation with the hand that is not being used to raise the lower extremities. It may also relieve pain due to muscle spasm in this area. Its principal value is in the possible assistance that may result from relaxation of muscle spasm, which in turn permits better localization of tender areas in the lumbar and lumbosacral regions, especially when soft-tissue structures are involved. However, since this maneuver may aggravate intrinsic, mechanical disease of the spinal column, it is not advisable to use it when an osseous spinal lesion is suspected. In doubtful instances, it is best to defer this maneuver until x-rays of this area have been obtained.

Passive Flexion of Knee.   This may aggravate pain in the lower part of the back and help to localize the site of pain, but it is not a specific test for any particular spinal or paraspinal lesion. The prone position and its resulting abdominal compression induce some degree of spinal hyperextension, which increases pressure in the subarachnoid space. It is thought by some to be more reliable for exclusion of protruded intervertebral disk than the straight-leg-raising test. Each extremity is tested separately and the knee is flexed as far as possible. When the knee is flexed fully to bring the heel to the buttock, disease in the lumbosacral region may cause pain and muscle spasm near the site of involvement. This maneuver may cause the pelvis or lumbar vertebrae to be lifted several centimeters or more off the table if the hips are partially flexed in an attempt to relieve the pain and muscle spasm.

Side Position

Compression of Iliac Crests.   This test is performed using firm, sustained downward pressure from the examiner's hands for about half a minute over the upper iliac crest on the side opposite from that on which the patient is lying. Pain produced in the region of the *sacroiliac joint* is a positive response that may be demonstrated by performing this test while the patient is lying on either the involved or uninvolved side. A positive response suggests sacroiliac localization of the condition, but a negative response (no localization of pain during pressure) does not exclude sacroiliac disease.

Sitting Position

Lumbar Spinal Motion. Examination of lumbar spinal motion when the patient is in the sitting position may reduce or eliminate any influence of the hip joints or hamstring muscles, and the findings obtained from tests carried out with the patient in this position can be compared with those obtained while the patient was standing. When the sacroiliac joints are abnormal, forward bending from the sitting position may be freer than that observed in the standing position because the gluteal and hamstring muscles, which also may be involved by the sacroiliac disease, are more relaxed. When there is an abnormality at the lumbosacral junction, diffuse muscle spasm, or spinal fusion, forward bending from the sitting position remains as limited as it was from the standing position. The interpretation of these findings is seldom precise, but sometimes these maneuvers may be of differential value.

Tests Referable to the Cervical Vertebrae. Raising the skull up from the neck by *manual traction* may be a helpful procedure for evaluation of symptoms in the region of the cervical vertebrae. The examiner stands in front of the seated patient and places the thenar eminence of each hand on each of the patient's cheeks just below the maxilla and the finger tips of each hand firmly against the occiput on each side. Upward and inward pressure is applied firmly, slowly, steadily, and equally with both hands. Maximal manual traction is achieved with about 10 to 20 kg pull but should always be painless. The examiner's pressure is then slowly released, and the patient's head is carefully permitted to resume its original position.

In an alternative technique for manual traction on the skull, the examiner performs the maneuver from behind the sitting patient. The examiner places his hands firmly on the sides of the patient's head with the fingertips under each mandible and the palms against the patient's ears and sides of the head. Upward pressure as just described is applied and then released slowly and carefully. With this technique, there is less of a tendency for the patient's head to extend on the neck in the course of the upward pressure; in either method, however, the examiner should control the relative straightness of the patient's head and neck. It is advisable to explain the test to the patient in advance in order to obtain better relaxation and a prompt response to a prearranged signal, such as having the patient raise a hand to indicate any unacceptable discomfort. These considerations help to insure the patient's cooperation, especially in the event of repetition of the test. Relief of possible radicular symptoms during manual traction suggests nerve root irritation at or near the intervertebral foramina, although muscle spasm also may be relieved temporarily by this maneuver.

Atlanto-axial subluxation may be indicated occasionally when movement or sliding of the first cervical vertebra back and forth on the second cervical vertebra is seen as a distinct jerk in the normally smooth movements of flexion and extension of the upper cervical part of the spine. This may be perceived at the same time by the patient as a feeling of irregularity or jerking (or described as a dull thump or clunk). Regularity or irregularity of movement between the atlas and the axis also may be evaluated by palpating the patient's occiput and the posterior aspect of the upper cervical part of the spine during flexion and extension of the neck. Another reliable indication of atlanto-axial subluxation is sometimes referred to as the *palate sign*. In this test the examiner slides the second (index) finger of one hand along the top of the patient's tongue until it touches the posterior pharyngeal wall. The examining finger is then moved up and down to detect a space between the anterior surface of the arch of the atlas and the body of the axis. The examiner's other hand is cupped around the patient's occiput to assist in flexion and extension of the neck while the examining finger palpates for abnormality in the relationship between these two vertebrae. Effective performance of this test is enhanced when the examiner has become familiar with the technique and the patient is able to tolerate and cooperate in the procedure. Atlanto-axial subluxation is usually the result of laxity of the transverse ligament of the first cervical vertebra due to inflammatory processes of rheumatoid arthritis or ankylosing spondylitis or to trauma.

Application of manual pressure to the top of a patient's head may reproduce or aggravate cervical radicular pain. It is more likely to reproduce the patient's symptoms if the pressure is applied while the patient's head is tilted toward the side of the involvement or when the neck is hyperextended. These maneuvers may be of differential value; however, it is advisable not to attempt them until an x-ray examination of the cervical vertebrae has excluded metastatic or osteoporotic disease of the vertebrae, subluxations or fractures of the cervical vertebrae or of the odontoid process or other bone, or cord lesions, which would contraindicate these procedures.

Precautions.   Subluxation of the atlanto-axial articulation may cause radicular pain extending into the occipital region or into the arms or may produce extrinsic pressure on the spinal cord with bizarre neurologic symptoms below this level. Pain may be aggravated by sudden head movements or when the vertebral column is jarred. The patient may also have some difficulty in restoring the head to its normal position after looking downward. Atlanto-axial subluxation will be apparent from x-rays of the cervical vertebrae including flexion and extension views, but when the symptoms described previously are present, manipulation of the neck must be avoided.

ADDITIONAL SPECIAL EXAMINATIONS

Digital Rectal Examination

This examination is an essential part of the examination of the back. It is performed best when the patient's hips are flexed, and this can be accomplished with the patient in either a comfortable prone position with knees flexed on the cushioned step of an examination table, legs and thighs abducted about 25 cm and hips flexed enough for the upper portions of the body to lie on the bed of the examination table, or in a supine Trendelenburg position with hips and knees flexed and lower extremities abducted. The latter position often is preferable for more extensive palpation of the sacrum, coccyx, and adjacent regions. The midportion of the sacroiliac joint lies just below and lateral to the promontory of the sacrum and often is palpable on the rectal examination. The lower aspect of the sacroiliac joint forms part of the upper edge of the sacrosciatic notch. Bimanual palpation of this region may be performed with the examiner's index finger in the rectum and the other hand placed externally over the lower portion of the back. Tenderness, if localized to the sacroiliac joint, may be more evident on internal palpation, but a marked discrepancy between tenderness palpated rectally and externally is unusual with sacroiliac involvement and should be noted if present. The examiner's finger in the rectum may be able to palpate sponginess or localize the presence of swelling or tenderness in the sacroiliac region on either side. Palpation of the sacroiliac area on rectal examination is limited by the proximity of the ischial tuberosities and thus is accomplished more satisfactorily in women than in men.

Palpation of Piriformis Muscle. It is also possible to palpate the piriformis muscle during rectal examination. The piriformis is a flat, pyramid-shaped muscle that arises from the front of the sacrum, where it is attached to portions of the first, second, third, and fourth sacral vertebrae, and passes out of the pelvis through the greater sciatic foramen on each side to become inserted into the upper border of each greater trochanter. Localized tenderness or spasm in this muscle may cause pain in the buttocks, and pressure over this muscle on rectal examination may produce definite pain and discomfort. A painful piriformis muscle also can be localized if the hip on the involved side is flexed and the knee is extended during the rectal examination.

Palpation of the Coccyx and Sacrococcyx. The coccyx and sacrococcyx are also examined by palpation rectally and bimanually as described for the sacroiliac joints. The coccyx may be manipulated by the finger in the rectum and the thumb outside to evaluate angulation and mobility and to localize tenderness on palpation or motion or both.

Palpation of the Symphysis Pubis

The symphysis pubis is a fibrocartilaginous articulation that has a thick mass of fibrocartilage called the interpubic disk. Although a sagittal cleft is often present in this disk in adults, the joint has no synovial lining. The disk is covered by heavy ligaments that connect the medial ends of the two pubic bones. The symphysis pubis is easily palpated externally in the midline at the base of the abdomen under the mons pubis. It may be moderately or markedly tender or slightly swollen, or both, in various forms of inflammatory arthritis such as ankylosing spondylitis, Reiter's syndrome, and in other types of osteitis pubis. Osteitis pubis is a painful condition of the symphysis pubis that usually develops after surgical procedures in adjacent areas, but it may occasionally be found without evident accompanying causes. In any event, it often is accompanied by resorption of the medial ends of the pubic bones, followed later by various degrees of reossification and usually by subsidence of symptoms. Tenderness, when present, can be compared to that which occurs with similar palpation of the manubriosternal or costochondral articulations or other bony prominences. The findings upon physical examination can be compared with those obtained by roentgenographic examination to help evaluate the clinical significance of the condition.

Bimanual Pelvic Examination

This examination is indicated in female patients to evaluate the lower spinal segments and the possible relation of pelvic organs thereto. The reader is referred to gynecologic texts for more details with regard to the technique of this examination. Backache is not commonly caused by disease of pelvic organs.

Neurologic Examination

Such an examination may be a necessary and integral part of the evaluation of the spinal column. The details of this examination can be found in neurologic texts and are beyond the scope of this publication.

SUGGESTED READING FOR ADDITIONAL INFORMATION

1. Rothman, RH, Simeone FA (editors): The Spine, Volumes I and II. Philadelphia, WB Saunders Company, 1975, 922 pp. (especially Chapters 7, 9, 13, and 14).
2. Farfan HF: Mechanical Disorders of the Low Back. Philadelphia, Lea & Febiger, 1973, 247 pp.
3. Jackson, R: The Cervical Syndrome. Fourth edition. Springfield, Ill. Charles C Thomas, 1978, 399 pp.
4. Schmorl G, Junghanns H: The Human Spine in Health and Disease. Second American edition by EF Besemann. New York, Grune & Stratton, Inc. 1971, 504 pp.
5. Mayo Clinic, Departments of Neurology and Physiology: Clinical Examinations in Neurology. Fourth edition. Philadelphia, WB Saunders Company, 1976, 385 pp.
6. Riseborough EJ, Herndon JH: Scoliosis and Other Deformities of the Axial Skeleton. Boston, Little, Brown and Company, 1975, 339 pp.

chapter **12**

The Hip

ESSENTIAL ANATOMY

The hip is classified as a spheroidal or ball-and-socket joint formed by the articulation of the rounded head of the femur with the cup-shaped cavity of the acetabulum. It is a weight-bearing joint that combines a wide range of motion with great stability. The hip joint has greater strength and stability but less mobility than the shoulder joint, which is also a ball-and-socket joint. Stability of the hip is due to (1) the deep insertion of the head of the femur into the acetabulum, (2) the strong fibrous articular capsule, and (3) the powerful muscles that pass over the joint and insert some distance below the head of the femur, thus providing considerable leverage for the femur and stabilization for the joint.

Acetabular Cavity

The acetabular cavity is formed by fusion of the ilium, ischium, and pubis. It is deepest and strongest superiorly and posteriorly, where it is subject to the greatest strain when a person is in the erect or stooped position. A mass of fat lies in the fossa at the bottom of the acetabulum. The acetabular cavity is deepened by a circular fibrocartilaginous rim, the glenoid labrum (or cotyloid ligament), that reduces the diameter of the acetabular outlet by forming a tight collar around the head of the femur and thus adds to the stability of the head of the femur in its socket. The lower portion of the labrum is incomplete, forming the acetabular notch. However, a transverse ligament over the acetabular notch completes the fibrous acetabular rim and converts the notch into a foramen through which blood vessels pass into the joint.

Articular Capsule and Ligaments

The hip joint has a strong, dense articular capsule that is attached proximally to the edge of the acetabulum, the glenoid labrum and the transverse ligament, which passes over the acetabular notch (Fig. 12–1). Distally, the capsule surrounds the neck of the femur and is attached anteriorly to the intertrochanteric line and posteriorly to the neck about 1.5 cm above the intertrochanteric crest. Thus, all of the anterior surface and the medial half of the posterior surface of the femoral neck are intra-capsular. Some of the capsular fibers are reflected upward from their femoral attachment and run along the neck of the femur as longitudinal bands or retinacula. The articular capsule is strong and thick over the upper and anterior portions of the joint; it becomes thinner and relatively weak over the lower and posterior portions of the joint.

The articular capsule is composed of circular and longitudinal fibers.

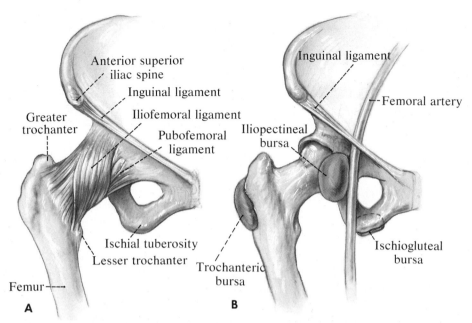

Figure 12–1. *A,* Diagram of the anterior aspect of the hip joint and adjacent bony structures. The fibers of the iliofemoral and pubofemoral ligaments fuse with those of the underlying articular capsule. The synovial membrane lines the inner surface of the articular capsule. *B.* Diagram of the relationship of distended iliopectineal, trochanteric, and ischiogluteal bursae (shown in blue) to the hip joint and adjacent structures.

The circular fibers are the deeper ones except over the lower and posterior portions of the capsule, where they appear near the surface. The longitudinal fibers are stronger and more numerous than the circular fibers and are divided into distinct bands or accessory ligaments that reinforce the capsule.

Iliofemoral Ligament. The iliofemoral ligament is the strongest and most important of the accessory bands. Crossing the front of the capsule, it extends from the ilium near the anterior inferior spine to the anterior portion of the base of the neck and intertrochanteric line of the femur (Fig. 12–1A). The lower portion of the iliofemoral ligament divides into two bands, forming an inverted Y shape. It is relaxed in flexion and taut in extension of the thigh and prevents excessive extension of the hip. In the upright position, the iliofemoral ligament keeps the pelvis from rolling backward on the femoral head and stabilizes the hip by pulling the femoral head firmly into its socket.

Pubofemoral and Ischiocapsular Ligaments. The pubofemoral and ischiocapsular ligaments are weaker than the iliofemoral ligament but help reinforce the posterior portion of the capsule. Respectively, they pass obliquely from the pubic and ischial portions of the acetabular rim to the femoral capsular attachment. Throughout their course they blend with the circular fibers of the capsule.

Ligamentum Teres. The ligamentum teres is an intracapsular ligament, that loosely attaches the femoral head to the lower portion of the acetabulum and adjacent ligaments. It has little effect on the normal motion or stability of the joint but is a channel for blood vessels to the head of the femur.

Iliotibial Band. The iliotibial band is a portion of the fascia lata of the thigh that extends inferiorly from the sacrum, the iliac crest, and the ramus and tuberosity of the ischium over the greater trochanter of the femur and lateral aspect of the thigh to insert into the lateral condyle of the femur, the lateral condyle of the tibia, the head of fibula, and the entire course of the lateral intermuscular septum that exists between the hamstring muscles and the vastus lateralis muscle. The significance of this structure is discussed in the section on "Special Tests for the Hip" on page 206.

Synovial Membrane

The synovial membrane of the hip lines the deep surface of the articular capsule. Proximally, it covers both surfaces of the cartilaginous rim of the acetabulum (glenoid labrum) and a mass of fat in the fossa at the bottom of the acetabulum. The synovial membrane also encloses the ligamentum teres in a sheath of synovial tissue. Distally, the synovial membrane is reflected upward from the femoral attachment of the capsule onto the neck of the femur and extends up to the cartilaginous surface of the femoral head. (Illustration of the synovial membrane of the hip has been omitted because this membrane is not palpable or visible on physical examination unless a rare synovial cyst of the hip is present.)

Bursae

Figure 12–1*B* shows the relationship of the iliopectineal, trochanteric, and ischiogluteal bursae to the joint and adjacent structures.

Iliopectineal Bursa. The iliopectineal bursa lies between the deep surface of the iliopsoas muscle and the anterior surface of the joint. It lies over the anterior portion of the articular capsule between the iliofemoral and pubofemoral ligaments and communicates with the joint cavity only in about 15 per cent of normal individuals.

Trochanteric Bursa. The trochanteric bursa is situated between the gluteus maximus muscle and the posterolateral surface of the greater trochanter. It is a large and usually multilocular bursa but is not palpable or visible unless distended.

Bursae also usually separate the deep surface of the gluteus maximus muscle from the tuberosity of the ischium and from the vastus lateralis muscle.

Ischiogluteal Bursa. The bursa over the ischial tuberosity is known as the ischiogluteal bursa. This bursa overlies the sciatic nerve and the posterior femoral cutaneous nerve.

Muscles

Principal Muscles of Motion. The hip joint is surrounded by powerful and well-balanced muscles that not only move the extremity but also help maintain the upright position of the trunk. Extension of the femur on the pelvis is performed by the gluteus maximus and hamstring muscles and the ischial head of the adductor magnus muscle. Flexion of the hip is carried out by the psoas major, iliacus, tensor fasciae latae, rectus femoris, sartorius, pectineus, adductores longus and brevis, and the anterior fibers of the glutei medius and minimus. Abduction is achieved by the glutei medius and minimus, and adduction by the adductores magnus, longus, and brevis, the pectineus, and the gracilis. Rotation of the thigh inward is performed by the gluteus minimus and the anterior fibers of the gluteus medius, the tensor fasciae latae, the adductor longus, adductor brevis, and adductor magnus, the pectineus, iliacus, and psoas major. Rotation of the thigh outward is effected by the posterior fibers of the gluteus medius, the piriformis, obturatorii externus and internus, gemelli superior and inferior, quadratus femoris, gluteus maximus, and sartorius.

Bony Landmarks

The bony landmarks of the pelvis will be described since the relationship of the pelvis to the femur is important in the evaluation of this joint (Fig. 12–1A). The crest of the ilium, the ischial tuberosity, and the greater trochanter are readily identifiable landmarks of the bony pelvis and femur. The entire iliac crest, which terminates anteriorly at the anterior superior spine and posteriorly at the posterior superior spine, is palpable subcutaneously.

The ischial tuberosity lies beneath the gluteus maximus and is easily felt when the hip is flexed because the tuberosity is then uncovered by muscle.

The greater trochanter of the femur normally lies the width of the subject's palm below the iliac crest about halfway between the ischial tuberosity and the anterior superior spine. It is located when the subject is in the erect position by finding a flattened depression on the upper lateral aspect of the thigh. In a thin subject the trochanter may produce a prominent projection on the surface of the skin when the hip is abducted and the thigh extended. This results from relaxation of the fascia lata by passive abduction of the thigh, allowing the upper portion of the trochanter to become defined more easily. If the hip is partially flexed and abducted by the examiner, the greater trochanter can be grasped between the fingers and the thumb, and easily outlined.

INSPECTION

Inspection includes evaluation of the patient's gait, functional and actual length of legs and length of thighs, body habitus, nutritional state, spinal curvatures, pelvic tilt, and scars of previous operations or trauma in the region of the hip.

Gait

Normal gait patterns vary widely. In healthy, normal gaits the abductor muscles of the weight-bearing extremity contract and hold either both sides of the pelvis level or the side of the pelvis not bearing the weight slightly raised. A "lazy" gait pattern is characterized by sagging of the nonweight-bearing side of the pelvis; an exaggerated swaying motion of the hips results during walking.

Several types of limp or abnormalities of gait are associated with disease of the hip. When the hip is painful or diseased, the body may tilt toward the involved hip and become balanced in this position by leaning to the affected side. This produces an antalgic gait and thrusts the weight of the body directly over the hip joint, decreasing the necessity for contraction of abductor muscles in order to hold the pelvis level and relieving muscle spasm to some extent. If the abductor muscles on the side of the involved hip become weak and are unable to hold the pelvis level when weight is borne on the involved hip, dropping of the pelvis on the side opposite the affected hip may occur and produce a Trendelenburg or abductor limp. The abductor limp causes the upper portion of the body to shift toward the normal side and decreases weight-bearing on the involved side. Both of these limps may be caused by a wide variety of lesions, and neither can be considered characteristic of any particular disease. Generally, diseases of the hip that cause pain tend to produce the antalgic limp, whereas diseases that produce an unstable hip and weakness of abductor muscles (such as poliomyelitis) tend to cause the Trendelenburg or abductor limp. However, either type of limp may be seen in patients with a painful hip or in those with abductor muscle weakness.

Abnormal Positions of the Femur in Relation to the Pelvis

Inspection of the relationship of the femur to the pelvis is of particular importance in the recognition of disease in the hip. Normally, the weight of the body in the upright position is supported equally by both hips, and the relationship of the femur to the pelvis is approximately the same on both sides. In the presence of unilateral disease of the hip, the weight of the body in the upright position is often supported mainly on the healthy leg, and in the standing position the leg on the involved side is usually placed in advance of the normal one because of flexion of the involved hip. This may be detected by having the patient stand erect and then alternate the body weight from one leg to the other. One side may be compared with the other by inquiring about the presence or absence of pain and noting disability or muscle spasm on each side in these positions.

Flexion of the Hip. Flexion is one of the most common findings on inspection that suggests abnormality of the hip. The flexed-hip position relaxes the articular capsule of the hip and tends to lessen pain, muscle spasm, and capsular distention. The patient with a flexion deformity of the hip frequently assumes a characteristic position when standing or lying supine on a flat surface. The spinal column is arched anteriorly in the lumbar region with production of lordosis and anterior pelvic tilt. This erroneously appears to reduce the flexion deformity of the hip. When the patient is lying supine on a flat surface, this compensatory pelvic tilt and lordotic curvature of the lumbar portion of the spinal column may allow the thigh to come into contact with the examining table (Fig. 12–2A). Extension of the flexed hip usually aggravates the pain in the hip by pulling taut the iliofemoral ligament over the anterior portion of the joint and thereby pressing the head of the femur firmly into the acetabulum. Flexion contracture of the hip also is indicated when the patient is lying prone and cannot extend the hip fully or when the examiner cannot lift the thigh into extension without simultaneously lifting the patient's pelvis.

Length of the Legs and Tilting of the Pelvis

Normally, when the patient is in the upright position the anterior superior iliac spines are level, and an imaginary line connecting them forms a right angle with each lower extremity. Apparent changes in the length of the leg may actually be due to lateral tilting of the pelvis associated with abduction or adduction deformities of the hip (see pp. 206, 207). If because of contractures one leg is in a position of adduction, the lower portion of that leg might cross the opposite normal leg. This position makes walking or weight bearing difficult or impossible. To compensate for this functional impasse, the pelvis is tilted upward on the side of the adducted thigh to help make both legs parallel for standing or walking. Elevation of the pelvis on the side of a fixed abduction deformity pulls the limb upward and makes it appear to be shorter than the other. On actual or bony measurement, however, the lower extremities are

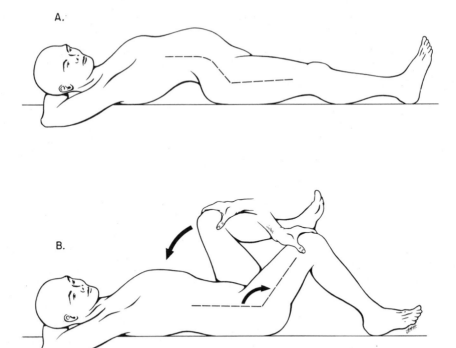

Figure 12–2. Diagram of the Thomas test for the detection of flexion deformity of the hip. See text for details. *A.* Flexion deformity of the hip is masked by an abnormal increase in the lumbar lordosis. *B.* Flexion of the opposite hip flattens the lumbar spine and reveals the extent of the flexion deformity in the hip.

equal or as nearly equal as is normal. To restore balance in the upright position and compensate for the apparent (functional) shortness of the leg, the patient may have to stand on the toes of the short leg or flex the knee on the normal side.

If one hip is held in abduction because of ankylosis or muscle spasm, the leg on the side of the abduction appears to be lengthened in the upright position. This causes an upward tilt of the pelvis on the normal side in an attempt to make the legs more nearly parallel for weight-bearing. The actual length of each leg measured from the anterior superior spine of the ilium to the medial malleolus is approximately equal, but measurements from the umbilicus to each medial malleolus would show apparent (functional) lengthening of the leg on the side of abduction.

Asymmetry of the Cutaneous Folds. Asymmetric positioning of the folds of skin in the popliteal or gluteal regions may give information as to the actual length of the leg and the femur when one side is compared with the other. Interpretation of the popliteal and gluteal folds is reliable only when the patient is standing with both legs parallel and both feet positioned firmly on the floor. In the presence of a pelvic tilt, the gluteal skin folds of the buttock will be higher on the side with the elevation of the pelvis than on the opposite side. Thus, if the left leg is actually longer than the right and the patient is standing with both feet on the floor, the gluteal folds on the left will be higher than those on the right. Elevation of the pelvis on the side with a fixed adduction deformity of the hip would also elevate the gluteal folds on the involved side, but the foot on this side would not be firmly on the floor. Asymmetry of the gluteal folds may also result from a gluteal abscess, muscle spasm, posterior dislocation of the hip, and atrophy or hypertrophy of gluteal muscles. When the popliteal creases are level and the patient is standing with both feet on the floor, the tibias and fibulas of the two legs below these creases are of equal length.

Either anterior or posterior dislocation of the hip causes a position of moderate flexion of the knee and hip. Anterior dislocation, however, produces external rotation and abduction of the hip. Posterior dislocation, which is the more common of the two, causes the hip to remain in a position of adduction and internal rotation. Fracture of the femoral neck is associated with acquired external rotation of the involved leg.

PALPATION

Before the examination by palpation is started, it is helpful to have the patient point out areas of pain or tenderness as specifically as possible. The common tendency of patients to do this with the fingers or hand hidden from direct view by the examiner should be avoided by having the patient stand with his back or side toward the examiner, or if the patient is being examined in bed, having the patient lie prone. When the muscles adjacent to the hip are relaxed to eliminate the pain of muscle spasm, pain referred from the hip arises from the attachments of the adductor muscles of the hip joint on the pubis and extends down the anterior and medial aspect of the thigh as far as the knee or arises in the groin in the region of the middle two thirds of the inguinal ligament, in the inferior portion of the buttock, and in the region of the greater trochanter. Sometimes the patient is unable to define the pain as superfical and can locate the area only as "deep" in the general region of the hip. Localization of pain to areas other than these may indicate involvement of structures other than those of the hip joint even though considered by the patient to be occurring in the hip.

After the patient has localized the area of pain or tenderness as specifically as possible, the examiner attempts to define the involved area more accurately by palpation, while noting soft-tissue swelling, tenderness, and superficial warmth where feasible.

Bony Landmarks

These have been described in the section on "Anatomy" (see p. 182).

Synovial Membrane

Synovial thickening or distention of the articular capsule from involvement of the hip usually cannot be palpated; rarely, a large quantity
of synovial fluid may produce palpable swelling and fullness over the
anterior portion of the capsule in the region of the iliopectineal bursa if
it communicates with the joint and has thereby accumulated some of the
fluid. It is difficult to differentiate involvement of the joint from tenderness of the soft-tissue structures overlying it. Occasionally, firm pressure
behind and somewhat superior to the greater trochanter may cause tenderness if synovitis or effusion is present, since the synovial membrane is
located relatively close to the surface in this area. Localized heat or
warmth in the region of the hip usually indicates soft-tissue inflammation
rather than disease of the hip joint because of the joint's deep location.

Disease of the hip, including synovitis, may be suggested by pain
in the region of the hip when the patient is supine and relaxed and the
examiner percusses the heel with his hand or fist while the patient's leg is
extended or when simultaneous firm pressure is applied by the examiner's
hands over each greater trochanter. *Percussion of the heel* and *trochanter-to-
trochanter pressure* are helpful methods of evaluating involvement of the
hip in a patient when examination is limited by the patient's inability to
assume an upright position.

Bursae

Iliopectineal Bursa. Fullness and tenderness of this bursa are
detected by palpable swelling and tenderness in the area of the middle
third of the inguinal ligament and lateral to the femoral pulse. The tenderness is aggravated by extension and reduced or relieved by flexion of
the hip. The possibility of a communication between this bursa and the
joint (present in 15 per cent of cases) has been mentioned. In this instance, extension of the hip increases tension of the fluid in the joint
cavity and its communication with the overlying bursa. Thus iliopectineal bursitis may represent either localized bursitis or extension of synovitis of the entire hip through the communication. The latter condition
also is described as a synovial cyst of the hip. The presence or absence of
a communication between a synovial cyst of the hip and the iliopectineal
bursa usually cannot be determined by physical examination. It may be
difficult to separate clinically iliopectineal bursitis from tendinitis of the
iliopsoas muscle, which lies superficial to the bursa (Fig. 12–1*B*).

Trochanteric Bursa. Trochanteric bursitis causes localized
swelling with tenderness on palpation over the greater trochanter of the
femur. Discrete localization of the swelling and tenderness by palpation
is the most important diagnostic finding of this condition. The pain is
usually aggravated by active abduction and rotation of the hip carried out

against the resistance of the examiner's counterforce, whereas flexion and extension cause relatively little discomfort. When swelling is not present, a purely bursal reaction may be confused with the more commonly encountered localized tendinitis or a painful reaction of a muscle attachment in proximity to the bursa and the trochanter. In the latter instances the absence of palpable swelling is particularly significant, for the site of tenderness often is noted on the posterolateral bony surfaces rather than over the bursa and the trochanter. It is difficult to differentiate between a purely bursal reaction and localized tendinitis in the region of the bursa. Careful localiziation of the tenderness by palpation of the bursal and adjacent areas usually is sufficient to permit this differentiation, as well as to distinguish it from the tenderness or referred pain resulting from involvement of the hip (Fig. 12–1B).

Ischiogluteal Bursa.   Tenderness over the ischial tuberosity may indicate ischiogluteal bursitis ("weavers' bottom") and sometimes is associated with swelling in this region. The swelling has been described as a circumscribed bulging area with a doughy feeling. In instances of acute ischiogluteal bursitis, the severity of the pain is a prominent feature, and it is aggravated by palpation. Tenderness over the ischial tuberosity also may be due to osteitis, irritation, or inflammation of tendinous attachments (Fig. 12–1B).

Other Findings in the Inguinal Region

The inguinal region should be carefully palpated for masses that might result from adenopathy, femoral or inguinal hernia, tumor, aneurysm, or psoas abscess.

MOVEMENT AND RANGE OF MOTION

The hip has a wide range of motion that permits flexion, extension, adduction, abduction, rotation, and circumduction. The angulation between the neck and shaft of the femur partially converts the angular movements of flexion, extension, adduction, and abduction into rotary movements of the femoral head within the acetabulum. When the hip is flexed and abducted, it loses much of the stability observed in the extended position, because then only a part of the femoral head is covered by the acetabulum, and the remaining portion is covered only by the articular capsule

Extension

Extension of the hip is defined as the upward (or backward) motion of the hip from the zero starting position, as shown in Figure 12–3.

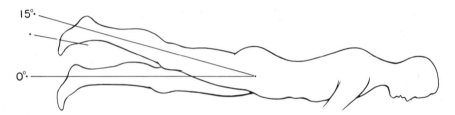

15°·

0°·

Figure 12–3. Diagram of normal range of extension of the hip with the pelvis and lumbar vertebrae stabilized. This range is determined with the patient in the prone position.

Motion beyond the neutral position (0 degrees) is sometimes alternatively referred to as "hyperextension." Whether such motion exists and if it does, to what degree, are still misunderstood and unsettled questions. The literature on this subject continues to be confusing and contradictory. Opinions vary from suggestions that there is no free range of extension to those that claim a normal range of extension of 30 to 40 degrees.

The crux of the dilemma is the technical difficulty of achieving the rigid stabilization of the pelvis required to avoid confusing extension of the hip with flexion of the opposite hip, compensatory lumbar lordosis, and downward or forward pelvic flexion, tilt, or rotation. Since such lumbar and pelvic motions may be slight, they are easily overlooked. Even when pelvic fixation is allegedly assured, an additional uncertainty exists about whether movement of the relatively bulky pelvic soft tissues is being confused with motion of the hip joint in extension. Thus, extension of the hip is likely to reflect some motion of the back, but this is relatively infrequent. Extension normally may measure 10 to 20 degrees less when the patient is prone or supine than when standing. This difference is attributed to a greater extensor torque created by the weight of the torso, which is centered slightly posterior to the hip joint in a normal standing position.

With the best available methods of eliminating exaggerated lumbar lordosis and accomplishing fixation of the pelvis, about 15 degrees of extension or hyperextension of the hip may be obtained (Fig. 12–3). With less adequate fixation or with abnormal laxity of ligaments of the hip (a rarity), the thigh may be hyperextended about 30 to 40 degrees.

In the usual method of clinical examination for extension of the hip, the patient is in the prone position and the examiner applies downward pressure over the sacrum with one of his flattened hands while lifting the thigh on the side being examined with his other hand placed about midway against the anterior aspect of the patient's thigh. However, this method of examination often does not effectively immobilize the pelvis and lumbar vertebrae. Better pelvic and lower lumbar fixation may be achieved with the patient supine with one hip and knee forcibly flexed and held in this position by the patient with his hands around his leg or ankle. This leaves both of the examiner's hands available for determining extension or hyperextension. The surface on which the patient is lying supine, however, limits the opportunity for detecting any extension. Furthermore, this may be a strenuous position for many patients, and it is not as practically applicable for determination of extension as for flexion deformity (see following section).

Some examiners recommend placing a small pillow under the abdomen of the patient in the prone position. The lower extremity is then moved in the direction of extension as shown in Figure 12–3, or while the knee is flexed to 90 degrees. An alternate method, which often is considered better, is also accomplished with the patient prone, with one extremity flexed over the end of the examining table to limit the possibility of pelvic or lumbar motion while the examiner attempts to extend the hip being examined (Fig. 12–4).

Measurement of extension (as well as flexion) of the hip also may be performed by using Nélaton's line* as a fixed line of reference on the pelvis, provided that the ischial tuberosities are equidistant from the midline (usually indicated by the location of the gluteal cleft) on both sides. The range of hip motion against this pelvifemoral angle is a downward and backward-opening angle of about 50 degrees in extension (and an upward angle of flexion of about 125 degrees), a net total or actual range of normal motion of about 75 degrees.

Measured against Nélaton's line, extension of the thigh is limited in the presence of a flexion contracture of the hip. The degree by which

---

*Nélaton's line extends on the same side of the pelvis from the anterior superior iliac spine to the most prominent part of the ischial tuberosity.

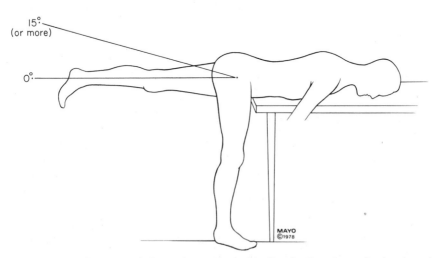

Figure 12–4. Diagram of alternative method of testing for the range of extension of the hip. Flexion of the opposite hip over the edge of the examining table with the patient in a prone position helps to stabilize the pelvis and lumbar vertebrae.

the pelvifemoral angle of extension exceeds the normal one of 50 degrees was considered by Milch to be the most clinically accurate method for determining the degrees of flexion contracture and one that can be employed regardless of any impairment in function of the lumbar vertebrae or the opposite hip.

Except for extension or hyperextension, motions of the hip are usually best determined with the patient in a supine position.

Flexion

The greatest degree of flexion of the hip is possible when the knee is also flexed. The thigh can be flexed to about 120 degrees from the neutral or extended position (0 degrees) if the knee has first been flexed to about 90 degrees (Fig. 12–5) and is held in this position by the examiner or by the active assistance of the patient. Sometimes the hip can be flexed until the anterior surface of the thigh presses against the anterior abdominal wall. If the knee cannot be flexed, flexion of the hip can be tested by raising the extended leg off the surface of the table. If the knee remains extended, tension of the hamstring muscles will limit flexion of the hip so that the angle between the thigh and the long axis of the body when the hip is normal may not be more than a right angle (90 degrees; Fig. 12–6). However, some individuals with apparently normal hips are only able to flex the hip to form an angle of about 75 degrees when the leg is extended, whereas in others the range of motion is much greater than 90 degrees.

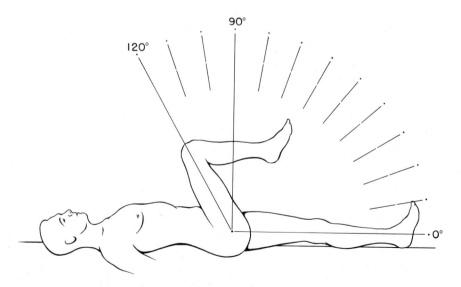

Figure 12–5. Range of flexion of the hip with the knee flexed.

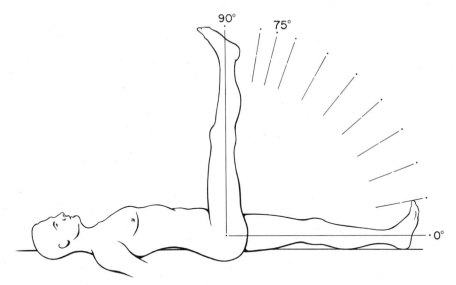

Figure 12–6. Range of flexion of the hip with the knee extended.

Exaggerated lumbar lordosis, if present, must be obliterated in order to determine the actual amount of limitation of extension or flexion deformity in the hip. This can be accomplished by forced flexion of the hip opposite from the one being examined while the patient is lying supine. When this forces the hip on the side being examined into a flexion deformity, the resulting maneuver, known as the Thomas test, is regarded as positive. This finding indicates restriction of extension in the hip (Fig. 12–2B). The degree of fixed flexion deformity can be estimated by measuring the angle between the involved thigh and the examining table. This estimate, however, is significantly inaccurate because pelvic fixation actually is incomplete, and the angle formed by the thigh being examined and the table is altered appreciably by motion of the thigh with respect to the pelvis and motion of the pelvis with respect to the table.

Abduction and Adduction

These movements are measured with both thighs and legs in an extended position and parallel to each other while the patient is supine. Measurement is made from the angle formed between an imaginary midline extended from the long axis of the body and the long axis of the leg. The amount of abduction permitted increases with flexion and decreases with extension of the hip. Normally, when the leg and thigh are extended, the hip abducts about 40 to 45 degrees from the neutral position before the pubofemoral and medial portions of the iliofemoral ligaments restrict it. There is, however, considerable variation in the range of ab-

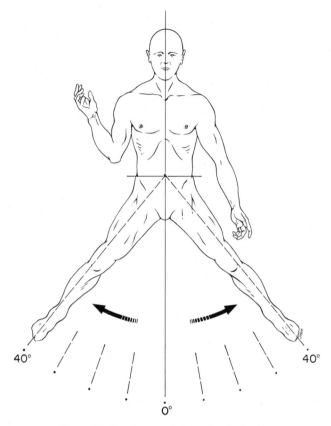

Figure 12–7.   Range of abduction in the hip.

duction beyond 45 degrees among normal individuals (Fig. 12–7). Limitation of abduction of the hip with the patient lying flat on his back is the most common limitation of hip motion found in the presence of disease of the hip. However, abduction of the hip also may be limited by spasm of the adductor muscles without involvement of the hip joint.

To test abduction of the hip, the examiner stands at the patient's feet, grasps the patient's extended left leg with the right hand and the patient's extended right leg with the left hand and abducts both hips simultaneously. This allows the examiner to detect minor degrees of limitation of motion by comparing one side with the other. With the patient's legs abducted, the examiner also can detect tilting of the pelvis by first abducting one of the legs and then the other while he observes the patient's pelvis to determine the point at which greater abduction is obtainable only by movement of the pelvis. Motion of the pelvis also may be detected in the course of unilateral testing of the range of abduction. For this, the examiner places one hand on the iliac crest of the side opposite to the one being tested or holds the opposite extremity at the

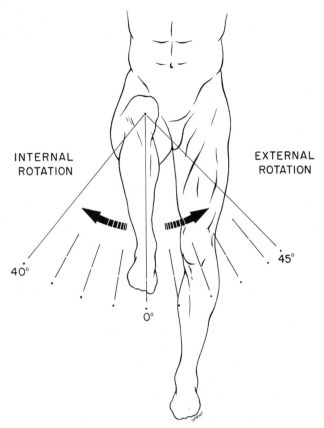

Figure 12-8. Range of internal and external rotation of the hip with the patient lying supine and with the hip flexed to 90 degrees on the side being examined while the other hip is extended. The examiner swings the foot inward for measurement of external rotation of the hip and outward for measurement of internal rotation of the hip. During this procedure the foot and thigh are moving in opposite directions. See text for details.

ankle, while watching carefully for the point at which pelvic motion begins.

Measurements with a steel tape of the distance between the internal malleoli (the "intermalleolar straddle") provide an index number for recognition of any changes that may occur from time to time in the total range of abduction of both hips. The normal range varies in different patients as a result of age and related or unrelated physical factors, such as the patient's height and physical agility.

Adduction with the leg straight normally is limited by the legs and thighs coming into contact with each other, but when it is possible to adduct the hip with enough flexion to permit crossing one leg over the other and then reversing the procedure, the degree of adduction of the hip of the extremity on top can be measured. Adduction then usually is possible to about 20 to 30 degrees from the neutral (starting) position.

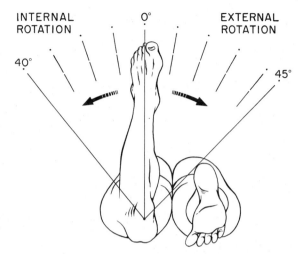

Figure 12–9. Range of internal and external rotation of the hip with the patient lying prone and with the hip extended fully (neutral position or 0 degrees) and the knee flexed to 90 degrees on the side being examined while both hip and knee are extended on the opposite side. The examiner swings the foot inward for measurement of external rotation of the hip and outward for measurement of internal rotation of the hip. During this procedure the foot and thigh are moving in opposite directions. See text for details.

Internal and External Rotation

These movements may be measured while the patient is supine with both hip and the knee flexed, while the examiner swings the foot inward or medially for measurement of external rotation of the hip and outward or laterally for measurement of internal rotation of the hip (Fig. 12–8). During this procedure the foot and the thigh are moving in opposite directions. The hip normally rotates inward about 40 degrees and outward about 45 degrees, but the range of rotation varies considerably among normal individuals, and both sides should be compared. External rotation is limited by the lateral band of the iliofemoral ligament; internal rotation is limited by the ischiocapsular ligament. Rotation of the hip increases with flexion and decreases with extension of the hip. Limitation of internal rotation of the hip is one of the earliest and most reliable signs of disease in the hip.

External and internal rotation of the hip can be tested with the patient's hip and knee fully extended while the patient is supine by rolling the thigh, leg, and foot outward and inward.

Rotation of the hip may be tested also when the patient is in the prone position; in this position the thighs and pelvis are well supported by the examining table. With this alternate method the patient's knee is flexed to 90 degrees by raising the foot and leg. The examiner then swings the foot inward for measurement of external rotation of the hip and outward for measurement of internal rotation of the hip while the thigh rests on the examining table (Fig. 12–9).

A further maneuver, that can be used when the examiner wishes to determine whether or not ankylosis is present can be made when the patient is lying supine. The examiner places one hand and forearm under the thigh on the side to be examined and supports the thigh on his forearm while the other hand is placed on the opposite iliac crest. The thigh is moved gently in various directions. In the presence of ankylosis of the hip the pelvis moves with each movement of the femur.

MUSCLE TESTING

Flexion. The prime movers in flexion of the hip are the psoas major (lumbar plexus, L2,3) and the iliacus (femoral nerve, L2,3) muscles. Accessory muscles are the rectus femoris, sartorius, tensor fasciae latae, pectineus, adductor brevis and adductor longus muscles and the oblique fibers of the adductor magnus muscle. Flexion of the hip is tested while the patient sits with his legs hanging over the edge of an examining table. The examiner immobilizes the pelvis by holding it with one hand over the ipsilateral iliac crest. The patient then flexes the hip through its range of motion while the examiner applies graded resistance proximal to the knee with his other hand, as shown in Figure 12–10. Flexion of the hip may also be tested while the patient is supine with the knee extended, but tension of the hamstring muscles when stretched may limit flexion and thus interfere with interpretation of the test performed in this manner. Substitution by the sartorius muscle (lumbar plexus, S1, 2) in flexion of the hip will cause lateral rotation and abduction of the thigh, and substitution by the tensor fasciae latae (superior gluteal nerve, L4, 5, S1) will cause medial rotation and adduction.

Extension. Prime movers in extension of the hip are the gluteus maximus (inferior gluteal nerve, L5, S1,2), semitendinosus (tibial branch of sciatic nerve, L4,5, S1,2), and semimembranosus (tibial branch of sciatic nerve, L5, S1,2) muscles and the long head of biceps femoris (tibial branch of sciatic nerve, S1,2,3) muscle. Extension of the hip is performed with the patient prone and the legs extended. The examiner holds the pelvis against the table with one hand by pressing down over the sacrum. The patient then extends the hip through its range of motion against the graded resistance provided by the examiner's other hand proximal to the knee.

Abduction. The gluteus medius muscle (superior gluteal nerve, L4,5, S1) is the prime mover in abduction of the hip. The gluteus minimus, tensor fasciae latae, and upper fibers of the gluteus maximus mus-

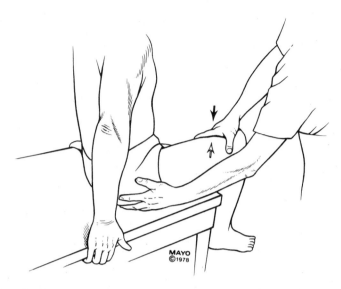

Figure 12–10. Test for flexors of the hip. In the sitting position the patient flexes the hip and helps immobilize the pelvis by holding the edge of the table. The examiner further stabilizes the pelvis with one hand and provides resistance to hip flexion with his other hand proximal to the knee.

cles are accessory to this motion. Abduction is tested with the patient lying on his side. The lower leg is slightly flexed at the hip and knee for balance. The upper leg is extended slightly posteriorly beyond the midline to avoid substitution by hip flexors. The examiner places one hand over the region of the superior iliac crest to stabilize the pelvis. The patient abducts the upper leg through the range of motion without rotating the hip, while graded resistance is provided by the examiner's other hand proximal to the knee, as shown in Figure 12–11. If the examiner fails to immobilize the pelvis, the patient may partially elevate the leg by strong contraction of the lateral muscles of the trunk, which move the pelvis.

Adduction. Prime movers in adduction of the hip are the adductor magnus (obturator and sciatic nerves, L3,4,5, S1), adductor brevis (obturator nerve, L3,4), adductor longus (obturator nerve, L3,4), pectineus (femoral nerve, L2,3,4, and occasionally obturator nerve, L3,4) and gracilis (obturator nerve, L3,4) muscles. Adduction is tested with the patient lying on his side with legs extended. The upper leg is supported by one of the examiner's hands in approximately 25 degrees of abduction. The patient then adducts the lower leg off the table toward the elevated leg without rotating the leg or tipping the pelvis, while graded resistance is applied by the examiner's other hand proximal to the knee joint, as shown in Figure 12–12.

Lateral Rotation. Prime movers in lateral rotation of the hip are

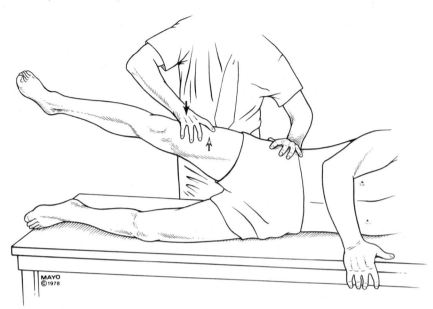

Figure 12–11. Test for abductors of the hip. The patient abducts the hip while the lower leg is slightly flexed at the hip and knee for balance and the upper leg is slightly extended. The examiner immobilizes the pelvis with one hand and provides resistance to abduction with the other hand proximal to the knee.

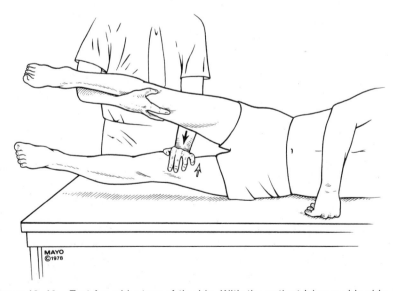

Figure 12–12. Test for adductors of the hip. With the patient lying on his side, the examiner supports the upper leg with one hand and arm. The patient then adducts the lower leg upward against the resistance provided by the examiner's other hand proximal to the knee.

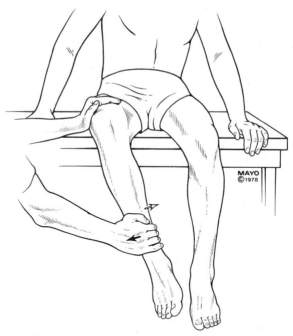

Figure 12–13. Test for lateral rotators of the hip. In the sitting position the patient rotates the thigh laterally and the lower leg medially. The examiner places one hand over the lateral aspect of the distal thigh to stabilize the leg and provides resistance to rotation with the other hand above the ankle.

the obturator externus (obturator nerve, L3,4), obturator internus (sacral plexus, L4,5, S1), piriformis (sacral plexus, S1,2), gemellus superior (sacral plexus, L5, S1,2), gemellus inferior (sacral plexus, L4,5, S1), and the gluteus maximus (inferior gluteal nerve, L5, S1,2) muscles. The sartorius muscle is accessory to this motion. Lateral rotation of the hip is tested while the patient sits with legs hanging over the edge of a table. The examiner places one hand over the lateral aspect of the thigh just above the knee to apply counterpressure to the thigh and prevent abduction and flexion of the hip, and the patient grasps the edges of the table to help stabilize the pelvis. The patient then rotates the hip and thigh laterally and the lower leg medially while the examiner applies graded resistance above the ankle with his other hand against the motion being tested, as shown in Figure 12–13.

  Medial Rotation.   Prime movers in medial rotation of the hip are the gluteus minimus (superior gluteal nerve, L4,5, S1) and the tensor fasciae latae (superior gluteal nerve, L4,5, S1) muscles. Anterior fibers of the gluteus medius, semitendinosus, and semimembranosus muscles are accessory to this motion. Medial rotation of the hip is tested while the patient sits with the legs over the edge of a table as for testing lateral rotation of the hip. The examiner uses one hand to apply counterpres-

sure over the medial aspect of the thigh above the knee to prevent adduction of the hip, and the patient holds on to the edges of the table to
help stabilize the pelvis. The patient then rotates the thigh medially and
the lower leg laterally, while the examiner provides graded resistance
above the ankle joint with his other hand.

SPECIAL TESTS FOR THE HIP

Heel-to-Knee Test or Fabere Sign

A simple test for detecting involvement of the hip joint without
differentiating the extent of limitation of a specific motion is the heel-to-
knee test, which involves to some extent several motions of the hip at
the same time (Fig. 12–14). The motions of the hip utilized in this test
are flexion, abduction, external rotation, and at the completion of the
test, extension. The initial letters of these motions were combined by

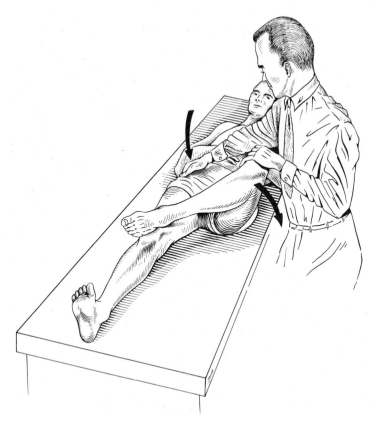

Figure 12–14. Heel-to-knee test or fabere sign for the detection of limitation of motion in the hip. See text for details.

Patrick to designate this test as "fabere sign." (The "f" is sometimes capitalized, but since this is not an eponymic designation, use of the lowercase letter is more appropriate.)

The hip and the knee on the side to be tested are flexed so that the heel lies beside or on top of the opposite extended knee. The hip being examined is then abducted and externally rotated as far as possible. The presence of pain, muscle spasm, or limitation of motion in the region of the hip on the side being examined constitutes a positive result of the test and suggests an abnormality of the hip. When this test gives a negative result, motion is normal and no pain or discomfort occurs, but some patients will describe discomfort in the lumbosacral region of the spinal column, which requires differentiation from the positive response. This test is performed easily and provides a general indication of hip disease but is less reliable for the detection of early disease of the hip than is specific measurement of internal rotation and abduction of the hip.

Measurement of Legs

This is performed most easily with the patient lying supine on a firm, level surface. The legs are extended, are parallel with the long axis of the body, and are parallel to each other. To prevent lateral tilting of the pelvis, the anterior superior iliac spines should lie on an imaginary line that is at a right angle to the long axis of the body. When marked scoliosis or severe muscle spasm is present, this may not be possible. The examiner then is alert to the fact that a pelvic tilt produces apparent and not actual shortening of the leg. The length of each leg is measured from the anterior superior iliac spine to the prominence of the medial malleolus on the same extremity. The measuring tape crosses the anterior surface of the patella at its middle. Comparison of the measurements of the two legs commonly reveals small differences in their length; a difference of less than 1 cm does not affect the gait. The significance of shortening in one leg is often difficult to evaluate. Shortness of one leg is often asymptomatic.

Difference in length of the legs can also be measured with an instrument consisting of two arms that rest firmly on the iliac crests and are attached to a housing on which a bubble level is mounted.* If the crest on one side is higher than on the other, the bubble deviates to the higher side. The amount of shortening on the opposite side is determined by placing boards of known thickness under the shorter leg until the bubble is centered. In cases of contracture of the lower extremity, only the apparent difference in length can be measured. In all instances, the procedure is accurate only if the pelvis is symmetric.

---

*Arch Phys Med Rehabil 53:45–46, 1972.

Shortening of the thigh may be detected by comparing the distances from the anterior superior iliac spine to the distal margin of the medial femoral condyle on the same side. If shortening is present, it may represent shortness or deformity of the femoral head and neck, shortness of the femoral shaft, or dislocation of the femoral head above the acetabulum. If the distances from the prominence of the greater trochanter to the prominence of the lateral femoral condyle are equal in both thighs, the shortening is not in the femoral shaft. An accurate or true measure of the leg length, however, needs to be determined by a scanogram that includes hip, knee, and ankle measured against a scale.

Tests for Congenital Dysplasia or Dislocation of the Hip

This condition may be detected in the following manner in infants: If the infant's hip is flexed to a right angle and then abducted, the lateral aspect of the thigh normally will reach or nearly touch the examining table or the surface on which the patient is lying and will form an angle of almost 180 degrees with the other thigh if both hips are placed in a similar position at the same time. If subluxation of one or both hips is present, abduction is distinctly limited, and the thigh will come only within 45 degrees or less of the examining table. Telescoping or up-and-down (cephalad-caudad) movement of the femur in relation to the pelvis may be demonstrable if the infant's hip is dislocated and the examiner alternately pushes upward and pulls downward on the thigh with the fingers of one hand behind the greater trochanter while the thumb is on the anterior superior iliac spine and the other hand grasps the patient's knee anteriorly. This maneuver should not be attempted when fracture of the hip is suspected.

Trendelenburg Test

Normally, when a patient bears the weight of the body on one lower extremity, the pelvis on the opposite side may be slightly raised by the contraction of the abductor muscles of the weight-bearing extremity in order to maintain balance. When this function is not normal owing to dislocation of the hip, nonunion of the femoral neck, coxa valga, or marked weakness of the hip abductors, all the patient's attempts to stand with the full weight of the body on the affected limb will cause the pelvis to drop on the opposite side, even with full cooperation of the patient, because of instability of the hip, lateral displacement of the femur, or lack of a stable fulcrum for the abductor muscles. The Trendelenburg test is positive when the pelvis drops on the side opposite to the weight-bearing extremity (see Gait, p. 186). This test is a measure of the patient's ability to use the abductor muscles of the hip properly regardless of whether the patient's habits of walking are good or bad.

Tests for Contraction of the Iliotibial Band

As noted earlier, the iliotibial band is a portion of the fascia lata of the thigh that extends inferiorly from the sacrum, the iliac crest, and the ramus and tuberosity of the ischium over the greater trochanter and lateral aspect of the thigh to insert into the lateral condyle of the femur, the lateral condyle of the tibia, the head of the fibula, and the entire course of the lateral intermuscular septum existing between the hamstring muscles and the vastus lateralis muscle.

The complete deformity resulting from contracture of the iliotibial band consists of flexion, abduction, and external rotation of the hip, genu valgum and flexion contracture of the knee, discrepancy in the length of the lower extremities, external torsion of the tibia on the femur, secondary equinovarus deformity of the foot, external torsion of the femur, obliquity of the pelvis, and increased lumbar lordosis. However, since the complete deformity is not always present in patients with contractures of the iliotibial band, the tests described next are helpful in detecting this disorder. Instability of the knee is currently a common, if not the most frequently encountered, factor to be evaluated in the presence of a contracted iliotibial band.

Abduction or Ober Test. The abduction test for contraction of the iliotibial band is performed with the patient lying on his side. The thigh nearest the table on which the patient is lying is actively or passively flexed until the lordotic curve of the spine is obliterated. The examiner then places one of his hands on the upper hip in the region of the greater trochanter, grasps the leg on the same (upper) side anteriorly and just below the knee with his other hand, flexes the knee to 90 degrees and fully abducts and extends the thigh. The examiner then slides his hand from its grasping position below the knee down the leg to grasp the ankle anteriorly. Under normal conditions this allows the uppermost thigh to drop down in adduction toward the table. When there is a contraction of the fascia lata or iliotibial band, the uppermost hip remains abducted and the leg does not drop back toward the table. In this situation, the iliotibial band can often be palpated easily as a rigid band in the subcutaneous tissues extending between the iliac crest and the anterior portion of the trochanter of the femur.

Adduction or Modified Thomas Test. The adduction test is another method for detection of contraction of the iliotibial band. This test is performed with the patient lying supine while the thigh opposite the side to be tested is held in forced flexion against the abdomen in order to stabilize the spinal column. The patient holds the thigh in forced flexion by clasping his hands together around his leg, while the other thigh and leg are tested by being extended or let down over the end of the examining table and then adducted. If the iliotibial band is contracted, adduction of the extended leg may produce a flexion contracture of the hip when the thigh is perpendicular to the level pelvis. If the flexion contracture of the hip is caused by tightening of the iliotibial band, it can be relieved by abduction of the hip. If the contracted iliotibial band does not produce a significant flexion contracture of the hip, it may be detected by attempting to adduct the extended leg on the side being examined. If the iliotibial band is contracted, adduction of the extended leg is limited to the extent that it is difficult or impossible to adduct the extended leg across the midline of the body; a partial abduction deformity of the hip is thus revealed by this maneuver. In addition, palpation of the contracted iliotibial band with the hip adducted or in a neutral position gives the feeling of a rigid band in the subcutaneous tissues extending between the iliac crest and the anterior portion of the femoral trochanter.

SUGGESTED READING FOR ADDITIONAL INFORMATION

1. Bombelli R: Osteoarthritis of the Hip. Pathogenesis and Consequent Therapy. New York, Springer-Verlag, 1976, 136 pp.
2. Tronzo RG (editor): Surgery of the Hip Joint. Philadelphia, Lea & Febiger, 1973, 840 pp. (especially Chapters 2, 3, 5, and 14).
3. Swartout R, Compere EL: Ischiogluteal bursitis. The pain in the arse. JAMA 227:551–552, 1974.
4. Renne JW: The iliotibial band friction syndrome. J Bone Joint Surg 57A:1110–1111, 1975.

chapter **13**

The Knee

ESSENTIAL ANATOMY

Joint, Articular Ligaments, and Menisci

The knee is the largest joint in the body. It is a compound condylar joint formed by three articulations which have a common articular cavity. One articulation is located between the lateral femoral and tibial condyles with its corresponding meniscus; another, similarly formed, is

208

situated between the medial femoral and tibial condyles with its corresponding meniscus; and the third lies between the patella and the femur. The fibula does not form part of the knee joint.

The bones of the knee are stabilized by articular ligaments. Ligaments of particular interest are the articular capsule, the ligamentum patellae, the medial (tibial) and lateral (fibular) collateral ligaments, and the anterior and posterior cruciate ligaments. The medial and lateral menisci are fibrocartilaginous disks found within the knee joint interposed between the femoral and tibial condyles.

The *articular capsule* is a thin, fibrous membrane that is strengthened by the fascia lata, tendons, and ligaments surrounding the joint. Anteriorly and superiorly beneath the quadriceps tendon, the articular capsule does not cover the synovial membrane. Fibers of the articular capsule and vertical fibers that arise from the condyles and from the sides of the intercondyloid fossa of the femur cover the synovial membrane of the posterior aspect of the suprapatellar pouch. Thus, the capsule lies on the side of, and anterior to, the cruciate ligaments. Distally, the capsule is connected to the borders of the menisci and then continues to an attachment on the straight margins of each of the tibial condyles.

The *ligamentum patellae* is the extension of the common tendon of the quadriceps that continues from the patella to the tibial tuberosity. A small, triangular fat pad, known as the infrapatellar fat pad, lies below the patella between the ligamentum patellae and the synovial membrane (Fig. 13–1) and may be more prominent at its protrusions on the medial and lateral aspects of the patella.

The *collateral ligaments* provide lateral and medial stability and support to the joint. The lateral collateral ligament is a strong, rounded, fibrous cord attached superiorly to the lateral femoral condyle and inferiorly to the lateral side of the fibular head. The medial collateral ligament is a broad, flat, membranous band attached proximally to the medial condyle of the femur just below the adductor tubercle and distally to the medial condyle of the tibia and to the medial surface of the tibia.

The two *cruciate ligaments* provide essential support to the anteroposterior plane. The anterior (medial) cruciate ligament is attached anteriorly to the intercondyloid eminence of the tibia and extends posteriorly and superiorly to the lateral femoral condyle on its medial and posterior portion. The anterior cruciate ligament keeps the tibia from moving forward on the femur. The posterior (lateral) cruciate ligament is attached to the posterior intercondyloid fossa of the tibia and to the posterior portion of the lateral meniscus. It passes superiorly and anteriorly to the medial femoral condyle on its lateral and anterior portion. The posterior cruciate ligament keeps the tibia from moving backward on the femur. Both cruciate ligaments also help to control rotation. The synovial membrane is reflected over the cruciate ligaments anteriorly.

The *medial and lateral menisci* are wedge-shaped, crescentic, fibrocartilaginous disks. The outside edge of each meniscus is thick and is

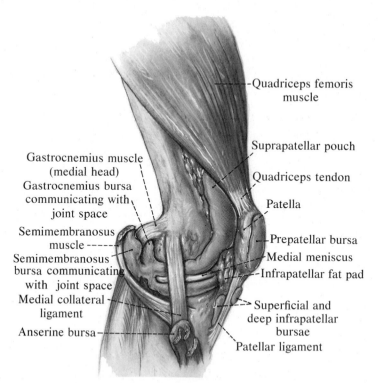

Figure 13–1. Medial aspect of knee showing distribution of synovial membrane and adjacent bursae when distended.

attached to the articular capsule. The inside edge is thin and unattached. The lateral meniscus is wider than the medial meniscus but is less thick at the outer margin. The inferior surfaces are flat and rest on the flat surface of the head of the tibia. The superior surfaces are concave and conform to the surfaces of the femoral condyles with which they come in contact.

Synovial Membrane and Adjacent Bursae

The synovial membrane of the knee is the largest in the body (Fig. 13–1). At the superior border of the patella, it forms a sac or pouch beneath the quadriceps femoris muscle on the anterior aspect of the femur. The suprapatellar reflection of the synovial membrane of the knee begins embryonically as a separate bursa; however, in most cases it communicates freely with the articular synovial space. Thus, it is appropriate to recognize this synovial reflection as the suprapatellar reflection or pouch of the knee rather than as a suprapatellar bursa. The superior reflection of the suprapatellar pouch normally extends as much as 6 cm above the superior pole of the patella.

On each side of the patella, the synovial membrane of the knee extends under the aponeuroses of the vastus medialis and vastus lateralis muscles, which are part of the quadriceps femoris group of muscles. The synovial membrane is somewhat more extensive on the medial aspect of the patella.

The region of the knee contains numerous bursae. Only the most constant and significant of these will be described (Figs. 13–1 to 13–3). A relatively large *prepatellar bursa* lies on the anterior aspect of the knee and separates the skin from the patella. A small *superficial infrapatellar bursa* is located between the skin and the proximal portion of the ligamentum patellae, and a deep *infrapatellar bursa* lies beneath the distal portion of the ligamentum patellae. Posteriorly, the *subpopliteal recess* is located on the lateral aspect of the joint and separates the tendon of the popliteus muscle from the lateral condyle of the femur; it is usually an extension from the synovial membrane of the knee joint. A *gastrocnemius bursa* lies on the posterior and lateral aspects of the joint between the lateral head of the gastrocnemius muscle and the articular capsule and usually communicates with the knee joint. *Another gastrocnemius bursa* is situated on the posterior and medial aspects of the joint between the medial head of the gastrocnemius muscle and the articular capsule; this bursa also usually communicates with the knee joint and with the semimembranosus bursa that lies superficial to it. The rather large *semimem-*

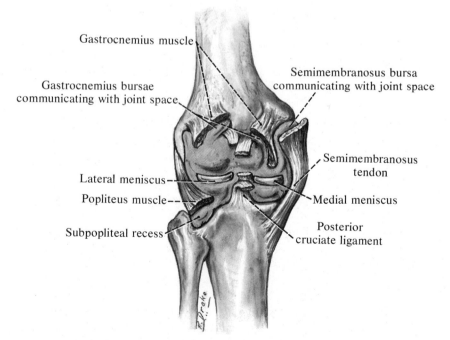

Figure 13–2. Posterior aspect of knee joint showing distribution of synovial membrane and adjacent bursae when distended.

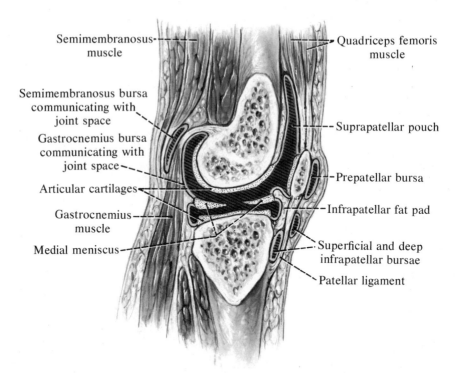

Semimembranosus-
muscle

Quadriceps femoris
muscle

Semimembranosus bursa
communicating with
joint space

Gastrocnemius bursa
communicating with
joint space

Suprapatellar pouch

Articular cartilages

Prepatellar bursa

Gastrocnemius
muscle

Infrapatellar fat pad

Medial meniscus

Superficial and deep
infrapatellar bursae

Patellar ligament

Figure 13–3. Schematic sagittal section of knee through area medial to midline show-ing relationship of synovial membrane and adjacent bursae to other joint structures.

branosus bursa is located posteriorly on the medial aspect of the knee. It lies between the semimembranosus muscle and the medial head of the gastrocnemius muscle. The *anserine bursa* is located on the medial aspect of the knee and lies between the medial collateral ligament and the tendons of the sartorius, gracilis, and semitendinosus muscles.

Muscles

Of the muscles that move and lend support to the knee, the *quadriceps femoris* is of particular importance. This muscle is the great extensor muscle of the leg and covers the anterior and lateral portions of the thigh. It has four heads that merge into a common tendon. The lateral portion is the vastus lateralis, and the medial portion is the vastus medialis. Between them are the vastus intermedius and the rectus femoris, the former lying beneath the latter. The common tendon of the quadriceps femoris continues distally to enclose the patella (the largest sesamoid bone in the body) as it passes over the knee joint to merge with the ligamentum patellae and inserts into the tibial tuberosity. Flexion of the leg on the thigh is performed mainly by the *hamstring muscles* (biceps femoris, semitendinosus, and semimembranosus), which are situated on the posterior aspect of the thigh. External rotation of the tibia and fibula on the femoral condyles is accomplished by the biceps femoris. Internal rotation of the tibia and fibula on the femoral condyles is accomplished primarily by the popliteus and semitendinosus muscles. The *gastrocnemius muscle,* which forms a large portion of the calf, helps to limit hyperextension of the knee and also plantar flexes the foot.

INSPECTION

The presence or absence of abnormalities of the skin, such as calluses, coarse thickening, rashes, or other dermal disorders, including infection, inflammation, psoriasis, and atrophy should be noted initially.

The knees should be observed for evidence of angulation deformity or instability both with and without weight-bearing. When lateral angulation of the tibiofemoral (knee) joint occurs, the condition is called "genu varum" (bowlegs; Fig. 13–4); medial angulation of the tibiofemoral joint is called "genu valgum" (knock knees; Fig. 13–5). Backward bowing of the knee ("genu recurvatum") results from hyperextension of the joint. When the knee cannot be extended fully, the angulation is described as a flexion contracture of the knee or as limitation of full extension of the knee. Observation of the range of motion and the manner in which the joint is used during ambulation may reveal a limp, hypermobility, con-

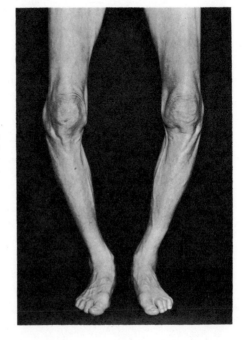

Figure 13–4. Marked instability and genu varum (bowlegs) of both knees in a patient with degenerative disease of the knees. Tenderness or pain occurs medially at the level of the tibiofemoral articulation.

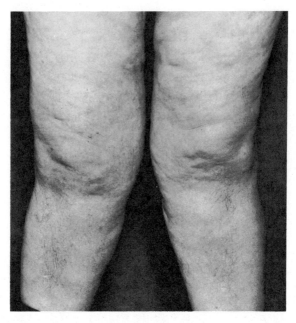

Figure 13–5. Genu valgum (knock knees) and degenerative disease of both knees. Tenderness or pain occurs laterally at the level of the tibiofemoral articulation.

tracture, sudden locking, or sudden buckling (giving way) of the knee. Locking is defined as a sudden or recurrent inability to extend the knee more than 20 to 25 degrees; usually it is accompanied by a painful and audible sensation variously described as a pop, click, snap, or catch that is aggravated by an attempt to achieve full, active extension of the joint. "Giving way," with or without pain, denotes weakness and instability indicative of ligamentous injury, although it may be observed as an induced behavioral response in emotionally unstable patients without any other evidence of joint weakness. In either instance, giving way needs to be differentiated from locking and popping. Movement and range of motion are discussed in more detail beginning on page 233.

The knees generally are inspected best with the patient relaxed and supine, with the knees extended as fully as possible. Some examiners prefer to inspect the knees first while the patient is in a sitting position with knees flexed to 90 degrees and legs hanging over the end or side of the examining table. A normal knee has distinct landmarks with concavities on each side of, and proximal to, the patella. These depressions tend to disappear, and outward bulging may even occur, in the presence of synovial thickening or effusion (Fig. 13–6). When the synovial membrane and articular capsule are distended by sufficient fluid, the knee may be held in a position of 15 to 20 degrees of flexion, since this position provides the synovial cavity with its maximal capacity to hold fluid and causes less discomfort from distention than any other position.

Synovitis of the knee is most obvious on inspection by the distention and swelling of the suprapatellar pouch. In such cases inspection may disclose abnormal fullness in the distal anterior portion of the thigh, which is often even more readily noticeable than the absence of the normal depressed contours adjacent to the patella. This fullness or swelling commonly extends to about 5 to 6 cm above the superior border of the patella, conforming to the extent of the anatomic reflection of this portion of the synovial membrane (Figs. 13–6 and 13–7).

Abnormal swelling in other locations adjacent to the knee should be differentiated from synovial thickening, effusion, or both. If the *prepatellar bursa* becomes distended, swelling develops on the anterior aspect of the knee between the patella and the overlying skin. Sharply demarcated margins usually indicate that the swelling is localized to the bursa and is not within the distribution of the synovial membrane of the knee. The skin overlying the prepatellar bursa may be shiny, atrophic, reddened, coarse, or thickened (Figs. 13–8 and 13–9).

Cystic *swellings of the menisci* may occur and typically are localized to the anteromedial or lateral regions of the joint space (Fig. 13–10). Such cysts arise more commonly on the lateral than on the medial aspect of the joint and are noted most readily with the knee flexed.

Swelling in the region of the popliteal space may be caused by distention of the semimembranosus bursa or the medial or lateral gastrocnemius bursa or by posterior herniation of the articular capsule and synovial membrane (Fig. 13–2). Distention of these structures produces a

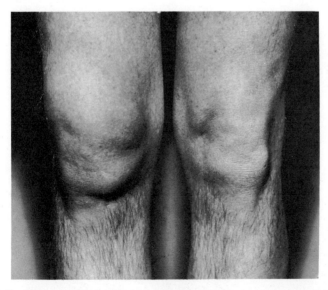

Figure 13–6. Mild synovitis (grade 1+) of right knee showing loss of normal contours and mild distention and fullness of suprapatellar pouch in a patient with rheumatoid arthritis. Note normal landmarks on left knee with depressed areas on each side of patella for comparison.

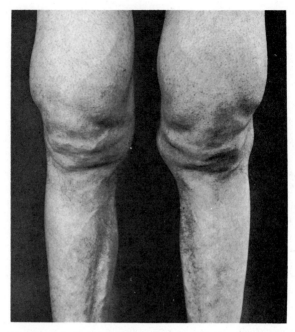

Figure 13–7. Marked synovitis (grade 4) of both knees of a patient with rheumatoid arthritis. Extensive fullness and swelling of the suprapatellar pouch are evident. Comparison of one knee with the other is made best with the patient supine and with both knees in the same degree of extension or flexion and as relaxed as possible.

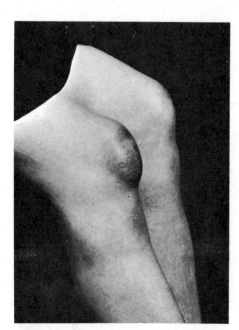

Figure 13–8. Prepatellar bursitis in the right knee, formerly called "house-maid's" or "nun's knee;" however, it occurs in males as well as females. The unaffected left knee is also seen in the background for comparison.

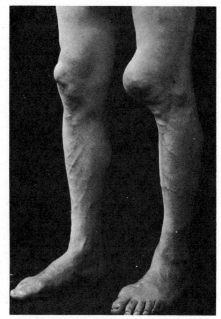

Figure 13–9. Tophaceous gout involving both knees with marked prepatellar bursitis on the left and mild prepatellar bursitis on the right. There is no evidence of synovitis in either knee.

popliteal bulge ("Baker's cyst"), which usually is an extension or herniation of the synovial membrane of the knee joint (see p. 226). Some popliteal cysts, especially those not resulting from inflammatory processes, appear not to have a definite lining of either synovial or other connective tissue cells. Distention of the semimembranosus bursa, which is situated posteriorly on the medial side of the knee, causes an ovoid swelling on the medial side of the popliteal space. This is more common in chronic inflammatory types of articular disorders.

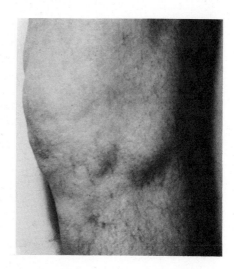

Figure 13–10. Cystic medial meniscus presenting as a 3 by 3 cm soft swelling along the midportion of the joint line of the right knee.

A popliteal cyst is usually more prominent with the knee extended or when the patient is standing and tends to become less tense and less prominent with the knee flexed. Flexion of the knee may be restricted by a popliteal cyst. Occasionally, a popliteal cyst may dissect downward into the calf muscles and produce an increased diameter and abnormal fullness of the middle or lower part of the leg (Fig. 13–11). Sometimes a popliteal cyst alone or its extension into the muscles of the calf may obstruct the veins or lymph vessels and cause swelling and dependent edema in the involved leg (Fig. 13–12). If the dissection or extension of the cyst occurs acutely, localized heat or redness, pain, and swelling may appear, and it may be necessary to distinguish the condition from phlebitis and cellulitis. Acute distention tends to occur when there has been a rupture of the popliteal cyst into the surrounding fascial spaces. A mechanical misuse of some type can often be identified as a cause in both acute and chronic development of popliteal cysts.

The anterior aspect of both thighs should be observed carefully for evidence of atrophy of the quadriceps femoris muscle. Atrophy in this muscle is a particularly significant finding, since the quadriceps femoris is the great extensor muscle of the knee and is essential for maintaining stability of this joint on weight-bearing. Atrophy of the quadriceps femoris commonly occurs in chronic disorders or with disuse of the knee. The medial (vastus medialis) portion of the quadriceps usually atrophies earliest; this change is easily overlooked since this portion of the quadriceps is relatively small. The vastus medialis is responsible for the final 10

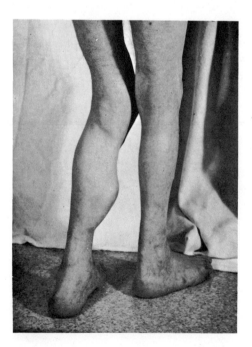

Figure 13–11. Extension of a popliteal cyst into the left leg of a patient with rheumatoid arthritis, producing a bulge in the inferior and medial aspects of the calf.

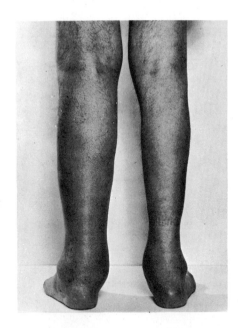

Figure 13–12. Popliteal cyst with secondary lymphedema of the left leg in a patient with rheumatoid arthritis. The cyst extends almost 18 cm into the muscles of the calf.

degrees of extension of the knee, and without its use the patient cannot maintain the knee in a completely extended position against gravity, nor can he walk with the knee straightened out unless the knee is locked in a position of maximal extension or hyperextension. Although atrophy of the quadriceps makes synovial effusion more evident, it also may give a misleading impression of the amount of enlargement of the knee (Figs. 13–13 and 13–14).

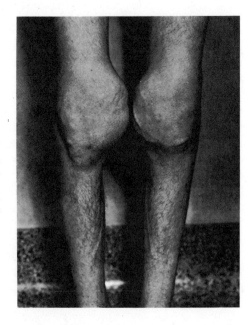

Figure 13–13. Marked synovitis of both knees (grade 3 on right and grade 2+ on left) of a patient with arthritis and chronic ulcerative colitis. More than the usual degree of medial pouching of the articular capsule and synovial membrane is evident, as is considerable atrophy of the quadriceps femoris and other muscles of the legs.

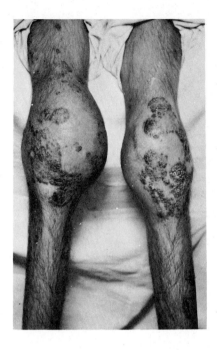

Figure 13–14. Psoriatic arthritis with extensive synovitis in both knees (grade 3 on right and grade 2− on left) and marked atrophy of muscles in the thighs and legs. The atrophy of the muscles creates an impression of exaggerated enlargement of the knees.

When it occurs, lateral dislocation of the patella is seen on full extension of the knee.

PALPATION

Whenever possible, it is advantageous to palpate the knee with the patient supine and the knee extended as completely as possible. If the quadriceps femoris muscle is not adequately relaxed, slight abnormalities in the underlying suprapatellar pouch or other portions of the synovial reflection cannot be palpated satisfactorily. Occasionally the examiner may prefer to palpate the knee when the patient is in a sitting position with the leg extended or the knee flexed a few degrees. For some patients this position may achieve greater relaxation of the leg and thigh muscles than is accomplished in the supine position. However, in this chapter, examination of each knee will be described from the patient's right side with the patient supine.

Synovial Membrane

Synovitis. For palpation of the suprapatellar pouch, the patient's hips should be abducted sufficiently to prevent contact of the knees, and the knees should be relaxed and extended as nearly to 0 degrees as possible. The examiner places his left hand lightly on the anterior aspect of the thigh about 10 cm above the superior border of the patella. The thumb is placed medially and the fingers are located laterally (for the left thigh) in a position that might be used to grasp the quadriceps muscle (Fig. 13–15). With the thumb and fingers exerting mild to moderate pressure, the examiner carefully palpates the underlying tissues as the hand is moved gradually toward the knee joint in an attempt to locate the superior edge of the synovial reflection of the suprapatellar pouch. The medial and lateral aspects of the quadriceps are palpated for swelling. As the soft tissues in this region are palpated under the fingers, the consistency, nodularity, thickness, warmth, and tenderness of the skin, subcutaneous tissue, and muscles are noted. If excess fluid is present, it is often helpful if the examiner's right hand is used to push superiorly any synovial fluid from the lower recesses of the synovial cavity to distend the suprapatellar pouch further and make it more easily palpable.

When a soft-tissue swelling with a somewhat different consistency from that of normal muscles and other soft tissues is palpated less than 10 cm above the knee in the manner just described, synovitis of the suprapatellar pouch is recognized. The swelling of synovitis and chronic synovial thickening seem fluctuant or "boggy" in comparison with the more solid consistency of muscles and adjacent soft tissues. The medial border of the suprapatellar pouch is particularly likely to be palpable, since it lies under the vastus medialis muscle, the first portion of the quadriceps femoris to become atrophied. Distention or thickening of the suprapatellar pouch may be caused by synovial thickening, synovial effusion, and tumors; areas of nodularity and induration alone or in combina-

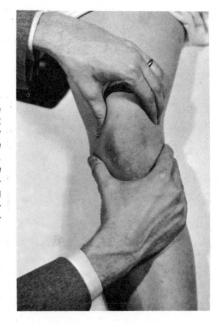

Figure 13–15. Palpation of the suprapatellar synovial pouch of the left knee. The examiner is standing on the patient's right side. The examiner's right hand firmly slides up from below and compresses the inferior portions of the synovial cavity. The right thumb and forefinger are over the medial and lateral joint spaces, respectively. The left thumb and fingers are palpating the lateral and medial borders of the suprapatellar synovial pouch. See text for details.

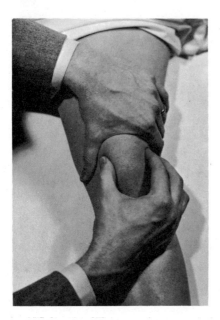

Figure 13–16. Palpation of the synovial membrane of the left knee. The examiner's left hand is compressing the suprapatellar pouch. The right thumb and forefinger are lightly palpating the space between the patella and joint proper for evidence of fluctuant distention. See text for details.

tion may be caused by fibrin masses, loose bodies, reaction from previous steroid or other intra-articular injections, and rarely in present-day clinical experience, tuberculoma. Since the suprapatellar pouch lies relatively close to the surface, the discovery of localized warmth and tenderness in this area also helps in the detection of significant inflammation of the synovial membrane.

In the next maneuver the examiner places his left hand just above the patella to compress the suprapatellar pouch firmly (Fig. 13–16). Compression of the suprapatellar pouch tends to force synovial fluid from the pouch into the inferior portions of the articular synovial cavity. As a result, the synovial membrane distends and is more easily palpable in regions adjacent to the articular cavity. While the examiner's left hand maintains pressure over the suprapatellar pouch, he places the right thumb medially and the fingers of the right hand laterally (for the left thigh and leg) between the patella and the tibiofemoral joint. This area is then palpated between the examining thumb and fingers for evidence of abnormal soft-tissue swelling or fluctuant distention of the articular capsule and synovial membrane. Care should be taken not to push the patella, fat pads, and adjacent soft tissues inferiorly or distally with the left hand, since this may produce a misleading impression of abnormal soft-tissue swelling in the area being palpated by the fingers and thumb of the right hand. Thickening or distention of the synovial membrane is palpated most easily on the medial aspect of the knee between the patella and the tibiofemoral joint space; normally the synovial membrane is not palpable in this area. A thickened synovial membrane has a "doughy" or "boggy" consistency and also may be fluctuant and accentuated if excessive synovial fluid is present.

Sometimes the margins of the synovial reflection can be palpated over the tibiofemoral joint space on the medial aspect of the knee just distal to the level of the midportion of the patella. The area available for palpation of the synovial membrane over the region of the joint space is relatively small; therefore, more experience is required to demonstrate synovitis here than in the suprapatellar area. Some rheumatologists consider the area over and superior to the tibiofemoral joint space on the medial aspect of the knee the most reliable site for the detection of mild synovitis and the differentiation of thickening and effusion of the knee joint. The articular capsule and synovial membrane can be palpated particularly well in this area because the overlying tissues are thin and the synovial membrane can be palpated against the adjacent bony structures. While the examiner's left hand is maintaining pressure over the suprapatellar pouch, the right hand in the same finger-thumb position as before is moved toward the articular space from a starting point about 5 cm distal to the inferior border of the patella. Again care should be taken to avoid pushing suprapatellar and infrapatellar soft tissues and fat pads distally when the suprapatellar pouch is being compressed, since these displaced tissues when palpated by the fingers of the right hand may give a misleading impression of synovitis. As the right hand is moved proximally, the thumb and fingers soon come to the tibiofemoral joint space, which is palpable when the patient is in the supine position as almost vertical grooves along the medial and lateral aspects of the knee. (See Figure 13–17 for positioning of the right thumb and forefinger on the

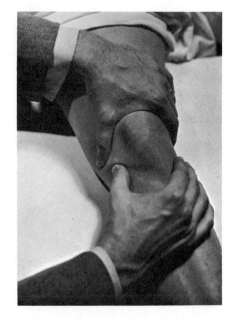

Figure 13–17. Palpation for synovial thickening and effusion over the medial aspect of the joint space of the left knee. The right thumb is palpating the medial part of the joint space. The left hand alternately applies and releases pressure on the suprapatellar pouch so that the right thumb on the joint space may detect any changes in synovial distention. See text for details.

medial and lateral aspects of the joint space, respectively.) If the synovial membrane is thickened or distended, its edges can be delineated over and superior to the region of the joint space and adjacent bony structures. Abnormalities of the synovial membrane are usually felt more easily over the medial aspect of the joint space, where the area of contact between the tibial and femoral portions of the joint and the weight-bearing surface is larger than over the lateral aspect of the articular space. The soft-tissue swelling of synovitis characteristically fans out sharply on the medial aspect of the knee with its apex facing posteriorly toward the joint space.

Figure 13–18 shows an alternate method of palpation for synovial thickening and effusion. The right hand compresses the suprapatellar pouch and the fingers of the left hand palpate the medial joint space.

Since the synovial fluid lies in a closed sac, compressing the fluid in the extreme limits of the synovial reflection over the region of the joint space, as described, causes the edge of the synovial membrane to become palpable as a bulge, which represents both the membrane and the movable fluid within the joint cavity. Such compression may cause or increase discomfort even before palpation over the area. If this bulge disappears following release of compression on the suprapatellar pouch, the palpable distention may be considered to have represented a synovial effusion; whereas, if it persists, it may be indicative of a thickened synovial membrane. Reliable differentiation between synovial thickening and articular effusion, however, is not always possible by the physical examination. Usually palpation is performed simultaneously for effusion and synovial thickening, and frequently both effusion and synovial thickening

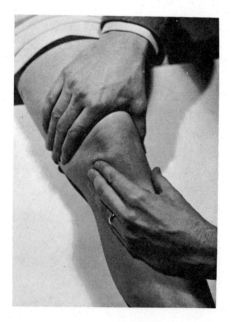

Figure 13–18. Palpation for synovial thickening and effusion over the medial aspect of the left knee using an alternate method of examination. The examiner is now on the patient's left side so that the left hand is comfortable while the fingers of the left hand carefully palpate the medial aspect of the joint space. The right hand alternately applies and releases pressure on the suprapatellar pouch. The fingers over the joint space may detect changes in synovial distention during this maneuver.

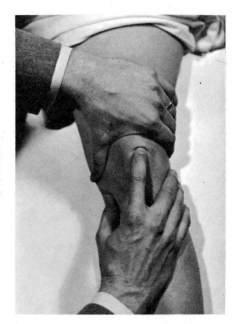

Figure 13–19. Palpation for effusion by ballottement of the patella of the left knee. The left hand is compressing the suprapatellar pouch. The right forefinger is used in ballottement of the patella in an anteroposterior direction.

are present in the same joint in inflammatory processes but not necessarily in other conditions. Palpation also is used to differentiate synovial thickening and effusion from muscle, lipoma or other adipose tissue, and inflammatory reactions of soft tissues, such as cellulitis. The differences in consistency are difficult to describe precisely but become appreciable through experience. Synovitis, already characterized as "doughy" or "boggy," simulates the feel of a liquid in a thin or thick plastic or rubbery bag when palpated, whereas muscle, adipose tissue, and cellulitis have differing consistencies but are more uniformly solid and less variably compressible.

Ballottement of the Patella. This may be possible when effusion is present, but to be successful it requires a relatively large amount of joint fluid and is not a sensitive method for the detection of a small quantity of fluid in the knee. To perform ballottement of the patella, the suprapatellar pouch is compressed with the examiner's left hand and the patella is pushed sharply against the femur in an anteroposterior direction with the forefinger of the examiner's right hand (Fig. 13–19).

Bulge Sign. Another maneuver that is most useful for the detection of minor degrees of effusion is referred to as the "bulge sign." For this examination the knee is extended fully while the patient is in a supine position with the muscles relaxed. The medial aspect of the knee is stroked and pressure is applied both proximally and laterally by one of the examiner's hands to express the synovial fluid from this area. The examiner then taps the lateral aspect of the knee with the other hand. A distinct fluid wave or bulge will appear soon afterward on the medial aspect of the knee between the patella and the femur if even a little fluid is present. It may be necessary to tap in several areas on the lateral aspect of the knee to localize the region that produces the maximal fluid wave, but the lateral aspect just above the midportion of the patella usually is the most effective site. Often this area can be localized sufficiently that pressure with only one or two fingertips causes a distinctly visible bulge on the medial aspect of the knee (Fig. 13–20). A reversal of this technique, accomplished by stroking the lateral aspect of the knee and tapping over the medial aspect, usually produces the same type of bulge, but synovial fluid may be less easily demonstrated using this method. The "bulge sign" maneuver reveals minor degrees of effusion, which often cannot be detected by other methods, and is most reliable when only a small amount of joint fluid is present (4 to 8 ml) and the synovial membrane is not detectably thickened. This maneuver has been attributed on some occasions to E. G. L. Bywaters, J. H. Kellgren, or P. Wood, but each has disclaimed originating the test in favor of a previous, unknown observer of the phenomenon. Thus, the term "bulge sign" has been used as a convenient and anonymous description of this physical finding.

Popliteal Space

The posterior aspect of the knee is palpated while the patient is prone, standing, or in both positions to detect or evaluate tenderness over the posteromedial portion of the popliteal space, the semimembranosus tendon, or the oblique popliteal ligament; tightness or spasm of the hamstring muscles; and a fluctuant synovial outpouching or cyst in the popliteal space. A synovial bulge in this area is also known as a "Baker's cyst" (see p. 217). When the lesion is sufficiently large, its cystic nature may be recognized by transillumination of the involved area. Such cysts may occur in patients with either rheumatoid or degenerative types of arthritis.

A popliteal cyst almost always communicates with the synovial cavity of the knee, although a synovial lining in the cyst is not always demonstrable. The cyst may fluctuate in size as fluid moves in and out of the joint cavity if the communication between the cyst and joint cavity remains ample and unobstructed. When the opening is very small (often 1 mm or less in diameter) or when the cystic fluid is very viscous or contains mucofibrin bodies ("rice bodies"), a communication may not be demonstrable even though it exists. Sometimes fluid can be compressed into the cyst from the synovial cavity but not the reverse. The ability to move the fluid either from anterior to posterior or vice versa indicates good communication. Compression of the suprapatellar pouch, with or without an accompanying pressure on the popliteal space, may distend a popliteal cyst to the point where its extension into the leg, if present,

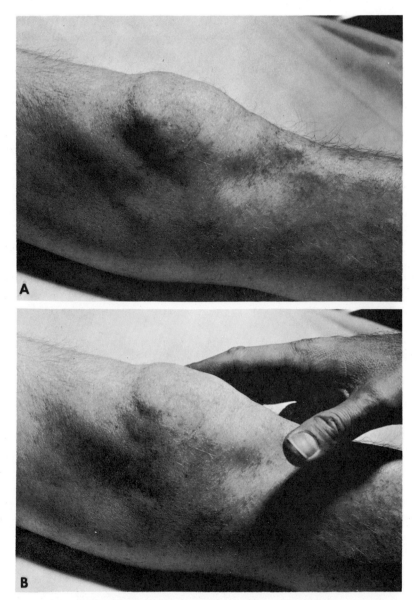

Figure 13–20. Bulge sign for demonstration of small synovial effusion of the knee. *A.* View of left knee from medial aspect showing depressed (shaded) area after this area has been stroked to move the synovial fluid out of this area, as described in the text. *B.* Same view showing bulge in the depressed area seen in *A* created by tapping lateral aspect of knee to move the synovial fluid back into the medial aspect of knee.

may easily be outlined by palpation and its lower edge delineated in the posterior or posteromedial aspect of the leg. All degrees of extension into the leg may be encountered; rarely, the dissection may extend as far as the Achilles tendon.

Examination of the leg may reveal an increased diameter of the calf at and above the level of the cystic extension. The cyst and adjacent areas may be tender, warm, or fluctuant on palpation, especially if the synovitis has resulted from an inflammatory process or has ruptured acutely into surrounding fascial spaces. The inflammatory reaction may simulate (temporarily, at least) cellulitis or phlebitis.

Although the presence of a popliteal cyst usually is determined best by palpation, its demonstrable connection with the anterior synovial compartments of the knee may be noted best or only by examination while the patient is supine with the knee extended and then partially flexed to release the tension of the iliotibial band, thus allowing deeper palpation. It is advisable to palpate the popliteal space both with the patient supine and the knee extended and also while the patient is standing, in order to localize the condition accurately.

Popliteal cysts, when localized to the popliteal space, may be differentiated from aneurysm by lack of pulsation. They also must be differentiated from fat pads, neoplasms, localized infections, and varicosities. A popliteal cyst may or may not disappear after anterior synovectomy.

Tibial and Femoral Articular Margins

The margins of the bones should be palpated for articular bony lipping or exostosis. Such spurs are palpable as irregular bony edges and often can be felt along the tibial or femoral margins of the knee joint. Pain at the joint line itself, when elicited on the medial side of the joint over the medial prominence of the femur, may indicate injury to the medial meniscus. This needs to be differentiated from involvement of the articular cartilage, the anterior cruciate ligament, or a combination thereof. Lateral tenderness at the joint line suggests involvement of the articular cartilage in that portion of the joint, the lateral collateral ligament, the iliotibial band, the head of the fibula, or combination thereof.

Bursae

The prepatellar bursa is easily palpable when distended, but certain other bursae in the region of the knee (for example, the anserine and the superficial and deep infrapatellar) are smaller and more difficult to recognize by palpation, even when tender or enlarged (Figs. 13–1 and 13–3). By localizing palpable swelling and tenderness to the region of the bursa rather than to the distribution of the synovial membrane, the examiner can differentiate bursal involvement from that of the articular synovial membrane. Thus, the reaction of anserine bursitis is restricted to the medial aspect of the knee and lies between the medial collateral ligament and the tendons of the sartorius, gracilis, and semitendinosus muscles. Prepatellar bursitis (housemaid's or nun's knee) is characterized by swelling and tenderness of the bursa that raises the skin over the anterior aspect of the patella (Fig. 13–8). When the bursa is markedly enlarged, prepatellar bursitis can simulate articular synovitis unless the bursal margins are carefully delineated by palpation. Both the bursal and synovial linings may be affected simultaneously, but by careful palpation the involvement of one may be distinguished from that of the other.

Infrapatellar Fat Pad

The infrapatellar fat pad lies beneath the patellar ligament, but when distended it is usually palpable as a soft-tissue fullness and tenderness on either or both sides of the patellar ligament (Figs. 13–1 and 13–3). Tenderness of the fat pad usually can be differentiated from involvement of adjacent structures by localization of such tenderness and swelling to the region of the fat pad.

Patella

Palpation of the patella may reveal several abnormalities. The patella is first palpated with the knee extended in the supine position and with the quadriceps femoris relaxed. The patella is pushed firmly downward against the femur by one hand of the examiner and then is moved about so that the articular surface of each quadrant of the patella comes into contact with the femur. Pain, tenderness, or grating that results from rubbing the patella against the femur indicates damage to the patellofemoral surfaces.

Crepitus or a grating sensation may be felt over the patella by the examiner when he holds his hands on it while the knee is flexed and extended either actively or passively or when the patella is moved while the knee is held by the examiner in either the extended or semiflexed position. Although patellofemoral crepitus is often associated with degenerative diseases of the knee, especially those involving the patellofemoral articulation, or with idiopathic chondromalacia of the patella, crepitus is often misleading and is of relatively little diagnostic value unless it is pronounced, since it is not uncommonly found in otherwise asymptomatic knees.

If grating sensations and tenderness noted during active flexion and extension of the knee are caused by abnormalities of the patellofemoral surfaces, these signs may disappear when the knee is moved passively by the examiner while attempting to hold the patella away from the femur. This maneuver is helpful in differentiating chondromalacia of the patella from changes in the tibiofemoral joint, for in the latter instance the grating or tenderness persists. Grating or crepitus also must be differentiated from popping.

Palpation of the undersurface of the patella may reveal tenderness if chondromalacia is present. To palpate the undersurface of the patella, the patella is displaced first to one side and then to the other. The amount of displacement possible varies considerably from one individual to another. Frequently, only the medial ridge of the undersurface of the patella can be felt. Tenderness that is present both while grating the patella against the femur and during palpation of the undersurface of the medial margin of the patella is significant if it is persistent and occurs in the same portion of the patella during both tests. Palpation of the portions of the vastus medialis mucle that insert along the medial and lateral borders of the patella may cause patellar pain that may be confused with other patellar disorders.

The patella plays a key role in the stability, motion, and strength of the knee. Dislocation of the patella is suggested when pain or tenderness extends beyond the area of the patellofemoral articulation to the medial retinaculum and parapatellar areas. A dislocated patella is tender on palpation and is displaced medially. It produces a knock-kneed appearance, and patients complain of a "click," a thud, or a sensation that the patella is slipping out of place during motion of the patella. (These sensations are sometimes erroneously confused with the popping of an injured meniscus.) The click is more likely to be felt than heard. Patellar symptoms and signs are most frequently elicited when the knee is flexed to 90 degrees from full extension or extended from 90 degrees to full extension, or both. This is to be differentiated from McMurray's test (p. 233).

Menisci and Collateral Ligaments

Tenderness localized to the medial or lateral aspect of the articular space between the condyles of the tibia and the femur suggests a tear or some other disorder of the meniscus. Other indications of injury to the meniscus include (1) limitation of extension or locking, each of which causes the patient to walk on his toes with the knee held at about 15 degrees of flexion, (2) a snapping or popping sensation inside the joint, and (3) local tenderness inside the knee toward the front of the joint or, when extension is attempted, along the articular line at the site of the injury. Other conditions that may simulate loss of extension include the presence of loose bodies, a torn anterior cruciate ligament that is displaced between the articulating surfaces, displacement of a condylar fracture, and spasm or contracture of the hamstring muscles. In the presence of spasm or contracture of these muscles, forced extension produces pain and tightness in the popliteal region of the knee. Tears or degenerative changes occur more frequently in the medial meniscus than in the lateral meniscus. Repeated examinations may be needed to determine whether a meniscus is the only structure involved. Occasionally, symptoms and signs of injury to the meniscus are found only or primarily at the compartment of the knee opposite the injury.

Tenderness along the ligamentous attachments over the medial or lateral femoral condyles extending above the region of the articular space, in contrast to the tenderness of injury to the meniscus, suggests a disorder of the collateral ligaments. Such tenderness, however, must be differentiated from tenderness of the fat pads of the lateral aspect of the iliotibial band, and of the biceps femoris and popliteal tendons. Turning the knee medially and putting slight stress on it will bring the lateral collateral ligament into prominence at the fibular head, with the popliteal tendon running just underneath it. The tensed iliotibial band is then palpable beneath the tendon. The iliotibial band is tightest at 15 to 30 degrees of flexion, and its distal portion is palpated best when the patient's leg is actively flexed (see page 206).

Sprains (tears of the ligamentous fibers of varying degrees, with or without joint instability) are the most common injuries of the knee because the ligaments have a finite limit to their elasticity; beyond that limit "something has to give." The medial collateral ligament is involved more frequently in sprains than the lateral ligament. The commonest site for a tear of the medial collateral ligament is at the medial prominence of the femur. The medial collateral ligament should be palpated to its distal attachment below and anteromedial to the joint line (Fig. 13–1). Rolling the palpating fingers over the leading edge of the medial line of the joint in search of a defect in the ligament can be a particularly informative part of the examination. Tenderness extending around the posteromedial capsule indicates additional injury to the medial compartment. Tearing of the lateral collateral ligament most often occurs at its attachment to the head of the fibula.

Lesions of the collateral ligaments may be differentiated from those of the menisci by abduction and adduction of the tibia with the femur stabilized. Complete relaxation of the extremity being tested is required in order to release the tensing mechanisms of the quadriceps muscles.

Abduction Test. The abduction test consists of a valgus strain applied to the lateral aspect of the knee joint by the examiner. The patient should be supine. The examiner grasps the lower part of the patient's thigh firmly on the anterolateral aspect to stabilize the lower end of the femur and prevent abduction of that bone. After stabilizing the femur and while the patient's knee is in complete extension, the examiner gently abducts the tibia with one hand by pulling the distal end of the patient's leg laterally. This maneuver tends to expand the medial aspect of the tibiofemoral joint, lessens pressure on the medial meniscus, and compresses the lateral meniscus of the knee. When this maneuver produces pain on the lateral aspect of the knee, the pain usually arises from the lateral meniscus or the lateral articular space. The same maneuver relaxes the lateral collateral ligament and tenses the medial collateral ligament. The test is repeated with the knee in 30 degrees of flexion, and the results from both the extension and partial flexion tests are compared for the two extremities. Thus, if the pain is felt on the medial aspect of the knee, it is usually due to the strain on the medial collateral ligament. Palpation usually can determine whether the area of maximal tenderness is over the medial femoral condyle or the joint.

Adduction Test. The adduction test consists of gently applying a varus strain to the medial aspect of the knee joint by using the examiner's hands as described for the abduction test, except that in this instance the pressure or stabilization is applied to the femur from the medial side of the knee being tested. The examiner adducts the tibia by pulling the distal end of the patient's leg inward. This tends to open the lateral aspect of the tibiofemoral joint and to compress the medial aspect. Because of ligamentous stretching, this maneuver produces pain on the lateral aspect of the knee if there is a lesion in the lateral collateral ligament; sometimes the point of maximal tenderness can be localized by palpation to the area adjacent to the lateral femoral condyle rather than over the joint space. Because of compression, this maneuver also may cause pain on the medial aspect of the joint if there is a lesion in the medial meniscus. The test is repeated with the knee in 30 degrees of flexion, and the results from both the extension and partial flexion tests are compared for the two extremities. Thus, while either the abduction or adduction test may produce pain in the presence of a disorder of a meniscus or collateral ligament, careful localization of the pain will often enable the examiner to differentiate a lesion of the meniscus from a disorder of the collateral ligament. Care is required when the knee is tested at only 15 degrees of flexion. An opening of the lateral aspect of the knee joint in that position could suggest injury to the anterior cruciate ligament and the posterior capsule, because both are tensed somewhat in flexion at that angle. A knee that is unstable both at full extension and at 30 degrees of flexion indicates a definite lesion involving a tear in the meniscus and injury of the anterior cruciate and collateral ligaments. These tests, however, are of more value in excluding a disorder of the collateral ligament than in excluding a tear in the meniscus.

Other Maneuvers or Tests. A variation of the abduction and adduction maneuvers can be performed by having the patient stand with his foot inverted and then placing a lift of solid material such as boards, books, or magazines about 2.5 to 4.0 cm in thickness under the medial side of the heel and sole. This increases the mechanical intra-articular pressure on the medial side of the knee in the region of the meniscus and also increases to a lesser extent the tendinous pull extra-articularly on the lateral side of the knee. With the patient standing on an everted foot, the reverse of this test can be performed.

Sometimes evidence of a tear in the posterior portion of either meniscus can be obtained as follows: The examiner places one hand over the anterior aspect of the fully flexed knee with the index finger flattened along the line of the joint on one side and the thumb on the other. The examiner then grasps the patient's leg at the ankle with his other hand and moves the knee repeatedly from full flexion to extension, at the same time rotating the leg medially and laterally. About 30 degrees of internal rotation and 15 degrees of external rotation can be expected on this maneuver. Significant anterior displacement when the leg is in 15 degrees of external rotation is positive evidence of injury to the capsular, medial collateral, and anterior cruciate ligaments. This maneuver, known as McMurray's sign, will often produce a palpable and sometimes audible snapping or pop when the torn meniscus moves in and out of place. When the click, snap, or pop occurs in the range of motion between full flexion and 90 degrees with internal or external rotational stress on the tibiofemoral joint, it is properly considered to be a positive McMurray's sign. A torn meniscus thus can be differentiated from patellofemoral abnormalities with grating or crepitation, which occur only in the range of motion from 90 degrees to full extension. McMurray's maneuver also may cause transient pain. A sudden click may be felt during active extension of the knee when the lateral meniscus is torn.

A torn or displaced lateral meniscus is also suggested when the audible sensation, however it may be described, results from squatting, rising from a squat, pivoting, or jumping. A torn meniscus is differentiated from a snapping popliteus tendon by the absence of a snapping sound when the tendon is tight or intact. A torn popliteus tendon usually cannot be distinguished clinically from a tear of the posterior horn of the lateral meniscus, since the precipitating injury frequently causes both. The McMurray test is the most important and most frequently used maneuver for evaluating a patient for internal derangement of the knee. Other tests have been proposed and can be found in orthopedic texts, but they are not usually of interest to, or used by, rheumatologists.

Cysts of the menisci (Fig. 13–10) may produce localized swelling and tenderness in the region of the joint space that is palpable between the tibial and femoral condyles medially or laterally, as described. These cysts usually arise on the lateral aspect of the joint and are noticed most easily when the knee is flexed.

MOVEMENT AND RANGE OF MOTION

The knee should normally extend to a straight line (0 degrees) and frequently can be hyperextended up to 15 degrees. The degree of extension is determined by measuring the angle formed between the thigh and the leg (Fig. 13–21).

The knee is then flexed passively by the examiner or actively by the patient, and the angle between the thigh and the leg is measured.

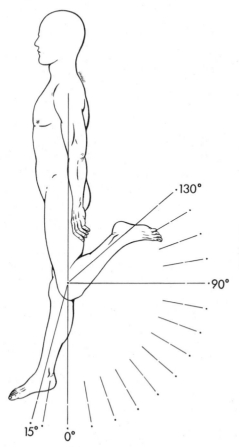

·130°

·90°

15°   0°

Figure 13–21. Range of flexion (0 to 130 degrees) and extension (0 to 15 degrees) of the knee. Flexion may reach 150 degrees in some people.

Normally, this angle of flexion ranges from 130 to 150 degrees (Fig. 13-21). A simple, useful, but less precise way of comparing flexion of both knees is by comparing the distance between the heel and the buttock when one or both knees are flexed as far as possible. Flexion contractures (limitation of extension) of the knee often complicate chronic involvement of this joint. Varying degrees of subluxation or dislocation of the knee are most often the result of posterior displacement of the tibia on the femur or occasionally from destruction of one condyle and supporting plate of the tibia. When as a result of such destruction the tibia is dislocated laterally or medially, abnormal lateral or medial mobility is present even though the range of flexion and extension of the knee is limited.

A catch or jerky motion sometimes can be felt or seen during passive flexion and extension of the knee when the joint space harbors loose bodies. On repetition of the motion the catch tends to occur at the same position on the arc of movement. The knee may lock or become fixed suddenly in partial extension while flexion from the point of limitation may remain relatively unrestricted. A catching or jerky motion also may result from the absence of both menisci because of surgical removal or from disintegration secondary to articular inflammatory diseases such as rheumatoid arthritis.

Stability

Two basic maneuvers will usually supply information concerning stability or ligamentous relaxation of the knee.

Collateral Ligaments.   Instability of the knee involves the collateral ligaments more frequently than the cruciate ligaments. The stability of the collateral ligaments may be evaluated in the following manner: With the patient supine and the knee in as close to zero degrees of extension as possible, the examiner fixes the femur with his left hand by grasping the lower anterolateral aspect around and under the knee while grasping the ankle anteriorly with his right hand; then he attempts to adduct and abduct the leg on the femur in a rocking fashion. Normally, there is practically no motion; increased mobility indicates relaxation or a tear of the medial or lateral collateral ligament. A loss of articular surface from a destructive process in the joint also may contribute to any instability revealed by this maneuver. If pain is elicited by this maneuver, it may indicate a lesion of a collateral ligament or a meniscus, as described under palpation (p. 230) or a lesion on the surface of the articulating cartilage. When the relaxed leg is passively flexed to 25 degrees and gentle stress is exerted on the medial compartment, characteristic "giving way" without significant springing back indicates complete disruption of the medial collateral ligament, posterior capsule, anterior cruciate ligament, medial meniscus, or any combination thereof. Lesser giving way to the same stress but with a definite spring back indicates an incomplete tear of the collateral ligament.

The knee should be observed for evidence of deformity and instability while the patient is standing. Weight-bearing on an unstable knee may disclose a considerable degree of genu valgum (knock knees) or genu varum (bowlegs), which may not be readily apparent from the manual maneuver described or when the knee does not bear weight.

Cruciate Ligaments.   A loud pop or snap at the time of injury is the hallmark of damage to the anterior cruciate ligament. Instability of the anterior or posterior cruciate ligaments may be detected as follows: The patient is examined in a sitting position with the knee flexed to 90 degrees and the hips flexed to 45 degrees. To stabilize the leg, the examiner sits on the distal portion of the foot of the extremity being tested while the foot is in a neutral position and places both hands on the patient's calf immediately below the knee of the same extremity with his fingers in the popliteal space and thumbs over the tibia. Because sitting on the patient's foot tenses the patient's hamstring muscles, some examiners prefer to stabilize the patient's extended or partially flexed leg by holding it between the examiner's lateral chest wall and forearm so that the patient's lower leg is in the examiner's axilla and the patient's foot extends posteriorly beyond the axilla. This technique is considered more reliable, since it can result in a positive test when other techniques do not. For optimal stability, when the right knee is being examined, the examiner places the patient's right leg just below his right axilla, and when the left knee is being examined he places the left leg just below his left axilla. This technique also allows the examiner to grasp the patient's knee with both hands.

To test the anterior cruciate ligament using either technique the examiner pulls the patient's leg toward himself and then pushes backward, repeating the same procedure on the patient's other leg to compare the findings. Normally, there is little or no excursion of the leg on the femur. A similar procedure with the examiner pushing the lower leg away from himself and then pulling it forward tests the integrity of the posterior cruciate ligament.

Abnormally increased forward excursion of the tibia on the femur indicates instability of the anterior cruciate ligament, whereas increased posterior mobility and excursion point to instability of the posterior cruciate ligament. Abnormal excursion of the leg on the femur during this maneuver is known as a positive "drawer sign" and is indicative of injury to the cruciate ligament. Absence of the drawer sign, however, does not exclude a tear in the cruciate ligament. A positive anterior drawer sign can be obscured when an anterior cruciate ligament is torn loose at its femoral attachment and becomes caught between the lateral femoral condyle and the tibial plateau.

Confirmation of anteroposterior instability thus demonstrated can be obtained by repeating the maneuver with the leg and thigh extended. Any anteroposterior movement in this position is abnormal. Anteroposterior movement when the knee is in the extended position is abnormal except for slight movement noted in some patients with thin legs. Some examiners prefer to perform this test first with the patient's leg and knee extended because it is less uncomfortable to the patient. If movement is present, the test is then repeated with the knee flexed. Hyperextension of the knee of more than about 5 degrees when the patient is supine also suggests injury to the posterior cruciate ligament, posterior capsule, oblique popliteal ligament or all three structures. Because the cruciate ligaments lie well inside the knee, they rarely are torn without injuries to more superficial ligamentous or cartilaginous structures.

MUSCLE TESTING

Flexion. The prime movers in flexion of the knee are the biceps femoris (sciatic nerve, tibial branch, S1,2,3 to the long head; peroneal branch, L4,5, S1,2 to the short head), semitendinosus (sciatic nerve, tibial branch, L4,5, S1,2,3), and semimembranosus (sciatic nerve, tibial branch, L4,5, S1,2,3) muscles. Accessory muscles to this motion are the popliteus, sartorius, gracilis, and gastrocnemius muscles. Flexion of the knee is tested best with the patient in a prone position with knees extended. The examiner places one hand over the lateral aspect of the pelvis to immobilize it and applies graded resistance just proximal to the ankle with the other hand as the patient flexes the knee through its range of motion. If knee flexion is performed with the ankle rotated laterally, the biceps femoris is tested more directly because it is placed in better alignment, as shown in Figure 13–22. If the ankle has been rotated medially, the semitendinosus and semimembranosus muscles are tested more directly during flexion. To prevent substitution by the gastrocnemius muscle, plantar flexion of the foot should not be allowed during knee flexion.

Extension. The prime mover in extension of the knee is the quadriceps femoris (rectus femoris, vastus intermedius, vastus medialis, vastus lateralis) muscle (femoral nerve, L2,3,4). Extension of the knee is

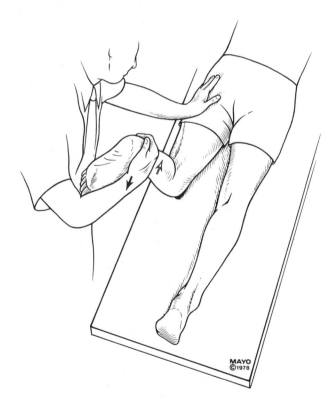

Figure 13–22. Test for biceps femoris muscle. In the prone position, the patient rotates the ankle laterally to put the biceps femoris in more direct alignment and then flexes the knee. The examiner stabilizes the pelvis with one hand and with the other hand holds the ankle in lateral rotation and provides resistance to flexion.

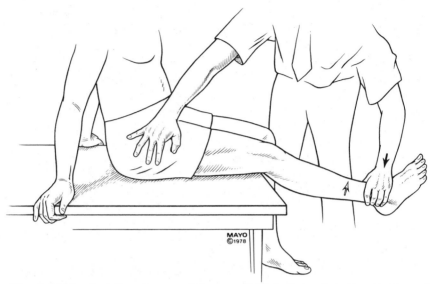

Figure 13–23. Test for extensors of the knee. With both hands behind him braced against the table the patient extends the knee. The examiner helps immobilize the pelvis with one hand over the upper lateral thigh and pelvis and provides resistance against extension with the other hand above the ankle.

tested while the patient sits with legs hanging over the edge of a table and both hands braced behind him. The examiner stabilizes the thigh by placing one hand over the pelvis or the proximal part of the thigh without exerting pressure over the origin of the rectus femoris or inducing pain. The patient then extends the knee through its range of motion while the examiner applies graded resistance with his other hand proximal to the ankle, as shown in Figure 13–23. Alternatively, quadriceps femoris weakness can be observed if the patient is not able to rise from a low chair (height less than 65 cm) or from a squatting to a standing position without using his hands or other supports.

SUGGESTED READING FOR ADDITIONAL INFORMATION

1. Helfet AJ: Disorders of the Knee. Philadelphia, JB Lippincott Company, 1974, 335 pp.
2. Smilliet IS: Diseases of the Knee Joint. New York, Longman, 1974, 459 pp.
3. Cailliet R: Knee Pain and Disability. Philadelphia, FA Davis Company, 1973, 149 pp.
4. Maquet PGJ: Biomechanics of the Knee: With Application to the Pathogenesis and the Surgical Treatment of Osteoarthritis. New York, Springer-Verlag, 1976, 230 pp.
5. Ricklin P, Ruttiman A, Del Buono MS: Meniscus Lesions: Practical Problems of Clinical Diagnosis, Arthrography and Therapy. New York, Grune & Stratton, 1971, 142 pp.
6. Renne JW: The iliotibial band friction syndrome. J Bone Joint Surg 57A:1110–1111, 1975.

chapter **14**

The Ankle and Foot

239

ESSENTIAL ANATOMY

The Ankle Joint

The ankle (talocrural) joint is a true hinge joint whose movement is limited almost entirely to plantar flexion and dorsiflexion. It is formed by the distal ends of the tibia and fibula and the proximal aspect of the body of the talus. The tibia forms the weight-bearing portion of the ankle joint. The fibula articulates on the side of the tibia but does not bear weight. The tibial and fibular malleoli extend downward beyond the roof or tibial portion of the joint and envelop the talus in a mortiselike fashion that gives lateral stability to the joint. The medial malleolus of the tibia projects inferiorly to articulate with the medial surface of the trochlea tali, and the lateral malleolus of the fibula projects inferiorly to articulate with the lateral surface of the trochlea tali (Fig. 14–1).

Articular Capsule, Synovial Membrane, and Ligaments of the Ankle

The articular capsule is lax and weak on the anterior and posterior aspects of the ankle joint but is tightly bound down by special ligaments on both sides (Figs. 14–1 to 14–4). Anteriorly in the midline the capsule extends from the tibia to a point approximately 1 cm distally on the neck of the talus. The articular capsule is less extensive posteriorly than anteriorly. The inner surface of the capsule is lined by synovial membrane. The synovial cavity of the ankle joint usually does not communicate with any other joints, bursae, or tendon sheaths in the region of the foot or ankle.

The strong medial and lateral ligaments of the ankle contribute to the lateral stability of the joint. The medial or deltoid ligament is the only ligament on the medial side of the ankle (Figs. 14–1 and 14–3). It is a strong, triangle-shaped, fibrous band that tends to resist eversion of the foot and may be torn in eversion sprains of the ankle. The lateral ligaments of the ankle consist of three distinct bands forming the posterior talofibular, the calcaneofibular, and the anterior talofibular ligaments (Figs. 14–2 and 14–3). These ligaments may be torn in inversion sprains of the ankle.

Tendons, Tendon Sheaths, and Retinacula Adjacent to the Ankle

All the tendons crossing the ankle joint lie superficial to the articular capsule and are enclosed for part of their course in synovial sheaths, which usually are about 8 cm long (Figs. 14–3 and 14–4). On the an-

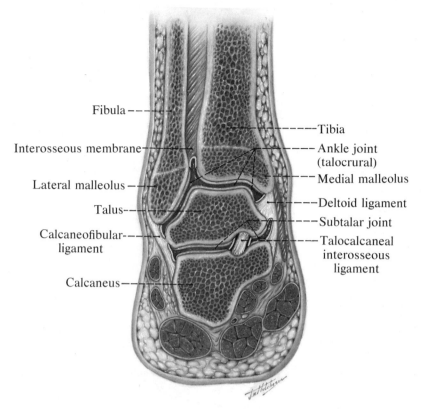

Figure 14-1. Frontal section through the ankle (talocrural) and subtalar joints. The distribution of the synovial membrane is indicated in blue.

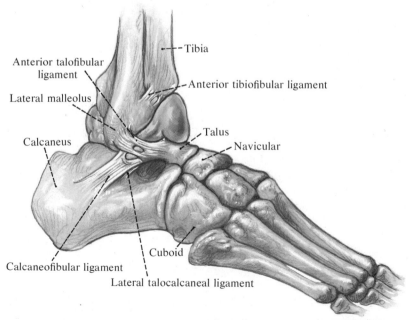

Figure 14-2. Lateral aspect of right ankle (talocrural) articulation showing the distribution of synovial membrane when distended.

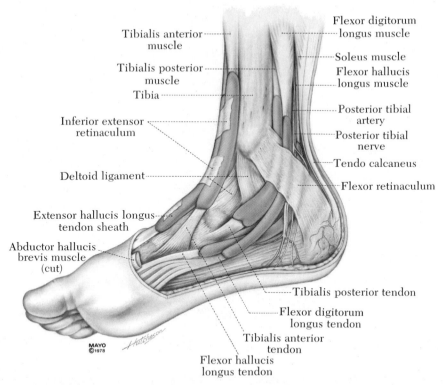

Tibialis anterior
muscle

Tibialis posterior
muscle

Tibia

Inferior extensor
retinaculum

Deltoid ligament

Extensor hallucis longus
tendon sheath

Abductor hallucis
brevis muscle
(cut)

Flexor digitorum
longus muscle

Soleus muscle

Flexor hallucis
longus muscle

Posterior tibial
artery

Posterior tibial
nerve

Tendo calcaneus

Flexor retinaculum

Tibialis posterior tendon

Flexor digitorum
longus tendon

Tibialis anterior
tendon

Flexor hallucis
longus tendon

MAYO
©1978

Figure 14–3. Medial aspect of the ankle showing the relationships of tendons, ligaments, and blood vessels. Tenosynovial membranes are indicated in blue.

terior aspect of the ankle the extensor tendons (tibialis anterior, extensor digitorum longus, peroneus tertius, extensor hallucis longus) and their synovial tendon sheaths overlie the articular capsule and synovial membrane. The tendons and tendon sheaths of the tibialis posterior, flexor digitorum longus, and flexor hallucis longus are located on the medial side of the ankle posteriorly and inferiorly to the medial malleolus; all three of these muscle tendons are plantar flexors and supinators of the foot. The tendon of the flexor hallucis longus is located more posteriorly than the other flexor tendons mentioned; it lies beneath the Achilles tendon for part of its course. The common tendon of the gastrocnemius and soleus (now designated as the tendo calcaneus but still commonly known as the Achilles tendon) is inserted into the posterior surface of the calcaneus where it is subject to external trauma, various inflammatory reactions, and irritation from bony spurs beneath it (Fig. 14–5). The Achilles tendon is separated from deeper structures by a pad of adipose tissue. The fibers of the small plantaris muscle unite in a narrow tendon that extends along the medial edge of the Achilles tendon to the posterior surface of the calcaneus. On the lateral aspect of the ankle, posterior and inferior to the lateral malleolus, a synovial sheath encloses the tendons of the peroneus longus and peroneus brevis; these muscle tendons

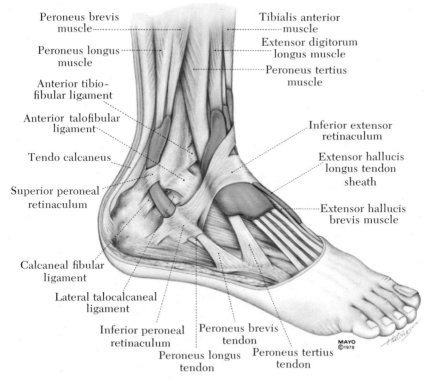

Figure 14–4. Lateral aspect of the ankle showing the relationship of tendons and ligaments. Tenosynovial membranes are indicated in blue.

extend the ankle on the leg (plantar flexion) and evert the foot. Each of the tendons or groups of tendons adjacent to the ankle may be involved separately in traumatic or disease processes.

Thickened fibrous bands hold down the tendons that cross the ankle in their passage to the foot. There are three sets of these fibrous bands or retinacula. The extensor retinaculum consists of a superior part (transverse crural ligament) in the anterior and inferior portions of the leg and an inferior part (cruciate ligament) on the proximal portion of the dorsum of the foot. The flexor retinaculum is a thickened fibrous band on the medial side of the ankle. The peroneal retinaculum forms two fibrous bands, a superior one and an inferior one, which bind down the tendons of the peroneus longus and peroneus brevis as they cross the lateral side of the ankle.

Intertarsal and Subtalar Joints and the Foot

The intertarsal joints provide additional mobility to the foot, since motion in the ankle is almost entirely limited to plantar flexion and dor-

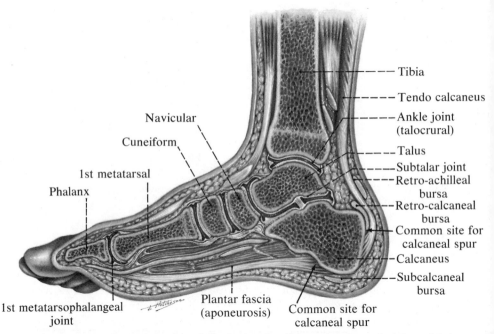

Figure 14–5. Sagittal section of the foot and ankle passing through the great toe. Common locations of bursae in the region of the heel are shown in blue and common sites for calcaneal spurs are shown by arrows.

siflexion. The intertarsal joints allow the foot to be inverted and adducted (supinated) or everted and abducted (pronated). Since the foot is arched, the weight of the body is transmitted anteriorly to the heads of the metatarsals and posteriorly to the calcaneus; these structures are the weight-bearing portions of the foot in contact with the ground. If the arch of the foot is to be adequately preserved during the strain of weight-bearing, the intertarsal joints must be firmly braced; consequently, the plantar surface of the foot is supported by unusually strong intertarsal ligaments that bind the tarsal bones together and prevent the arch of the foot from collapsing. The arch of the foot and the tarsal bones are supported also by the plantar aponeurosis, the short muscles of the foot, and long tendons that cross the ankle in their passsage into the sole of the foot.

Subtalar Joint. The subtalar (subastragalar) joint is a particularly important intertarsal joint, since it permits inversion and eversion of the foot. Sometimes the term "subtalar joint" is used to refer to the talocalcaneal joint or the posterior articulation between the talus and the calcaneus. However, as the term is used clinically, the subtalar joint is a functional unit that includes not only the posterior talocalcaneal joint but also the talocalcaneal portion of the talocalcaneonavicular joint and the talocalcaneal interosseous ligament that lies between these joints. The articular capsule and synovial membrane of this joint are tightly bound to the bones composing the joint and allow little if any distention of the articular cavity. Thus, the "subtalar joint" describes the total articulation between the talus and the calcaneus and is responsible for most of the motions of inversion and eversion of the foot (Figs. 14–1 and 14–2). Balance in walking and in more skilled or physically stressful activities is accomplished by coordination of all the muscles controlling the ankle; none of these muscles insert on the talus.

The relative lengths of the first and second metatarsal bones are variable. Ordinarily the first and second metatarsals are about the same length or the second metatarsal is shorter than the first. However, in some individuals the second metatarsal may be longer than the first. Shortness of the first metatarsal bone tends to be hereditary and is usually present in the atavistic type of foot. A short or unstable first metatarsal bone tends to place additional strain on the second metatarsal and adjacent structures in the mid-tarsal area and to subject the second metatarsal and mid-portion of the foot to added trauma. This may be of significance in predisposing the foot to disorders of the longitudinal arch and fore part of the foot and also may make the second and third metatarsals susceptible to injury such as march fractures.

The plantar aponeurosis or fascia is a fibrous structure of great strength that extends from the calcaneus forward as a relatively narrow band and then divides at about the middle of the foot into portions for each of the five toes. The plantar aponeurosis becomes thinner as it extends distally in a fashion similar to that of the palmar aponeurosis in the hand and fingers. The area of the plantar aponeurosis near the attachment of the plantar fascia to the calcaneus is particularly subject to the effects of trauma, inflammatory reactions, and bony spur formation (Fig. 14–5).

Metatarsophalangeal and Interphalangeal Joints

The anatomy of the metatarsophalangeal joints and the proximal and distal interphalangeal joints of the foot closely resembles the anatomy of the corresponding joints in the hand (see pp. 112–114). Each of these joints has an articular capsule lined with synovial membrane. The extensor tendon completes the capsule dorsally, the collateral ligaments strengthen the capsule on its sides, and plantar ligaments support the plantar portion of the capsule. The metatarsophalangeal joints normally undergo little flexion, and the articular capsules and synovial membranes are tighter than they are over the corresponding metacarpophalangeal joints in the hand.

Bursae

The largest bursae in the foot are commonly adjacent to the first and fifth metatarsophalangeal joints and about the heel. The bursae about the heel are likely to occur in three locations: (1) between the skin and the Achilles tendon, (2) between the Achilles tendon and the posterior aspect of the calcaneus, and (3) between the skin on the sole of the foot and the plantar surface of the calcaneus at the attachment of the plantar fascia (Fig. 14–5). Subcutaneous bursae are likely to develop in areas that are subject to most of the abnormal weight-bearing or friction. Thus, a bursal reaction may form between the thickened skin (callus) and the underlying bony prominence of the first metatarsal head in a hallux valgus deformity of the great toe or under the callus over the prominence of a proximal interphalangeal joint in a hammer toe deformity.

INSPECTION

The foot and the ankle are observed while the patient is standing, walking, and in a nonweight-bearing position. Both feet and ankles are compared anteriorly, posteriorly, and from the sides for evidence of swelling and atrophy, deformities of the foot and toes, location of calluses and bursal reactions, subcutaneous nodules, cutaneous changes, edema, and appearance of the nails (Figs. 14–6 through 14–12). It is helpful to note the location of calluses and bursal reactions in the foot,

Text continued on page 250.

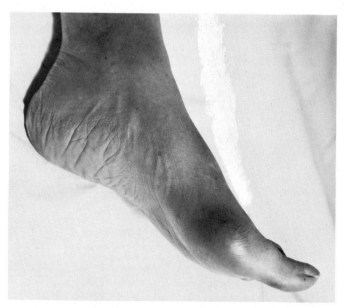

Figure 14–6. Acute gouty arthritis with maximal reaction over the medial aspect of the first metatarsophalangeal joint. The involved area extends well beyond the joint proper and exhibits all the manifestations of acute inflammation: swelling, red discoloration, heat, and exquisite tenderness.

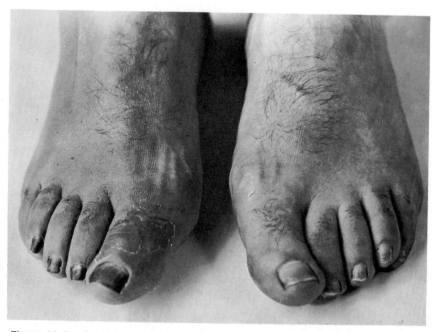

Figure 14–7. Subsiding attack of acute gouty arthritis in the interphalangeal joint of the right first toe. The skin over the affected area is desquamating.

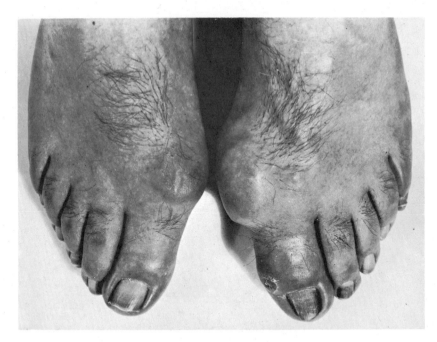

Figure 14–8. Large tophus over region of the metatarsophalangeal joint of the left first toe in a patient with chronic tophaceous gout.

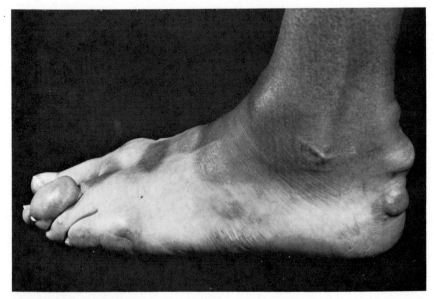

Figure 14–9. Tophi over the region of the Achilles tendon and in the third toe due to chronic tophaceous gout.

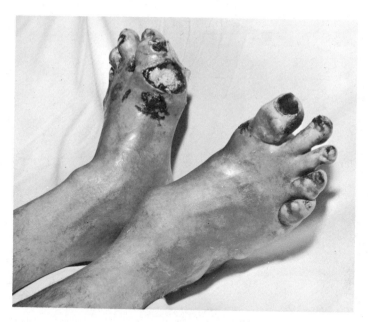

Figure 14–10. Advanced tophaceous gout with ulcerations of skin overlying deposits of urate and areas of necrosis. Modern treatment has made such extensive changes rare.

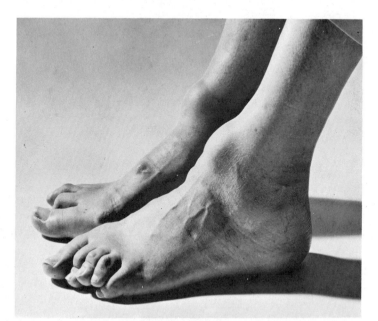

Figure 14–11. Synovial bulge (sometimes referred to as a synovial cyst) on the anterior aspect of both ankles in a patient with rheumatoid arthritis. The cyst in each ankle communicates with the joint cavity and represents a visible distention of the synovial membrane of the joint. Hammer-toe deformities in both feet are also present and the toes do not touch the floor surface because of the deformity and the swelling of the affected metatarsophalangeal joints.

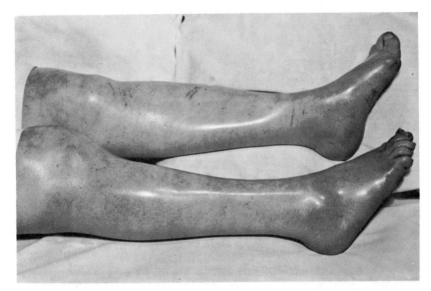

Figure 14-12. Bilateral equinus position of the feet in a bedridden patient with rheumatoid arthritis. Contractures of the Achilles tendons have drawn the heels cephalad and caused plantar flexion of the feet. Prolonged disuse has also resulted in shiny and atrophic skin of the legs.

since their presence indicates areas of abnormal pressure or friction as described. In deformed feet, calluses and bursal reactions may occur in unusual positions, corresponding to the location of pressure points. Examination of well-worn shoes also helps to illustrate how the patient walks.

Swelling in Joints of Foot and Ankle and Adjacent Structures

Effusion or synovial swelling involving the ankle (talocrural) joint is most likely to cause swelling or fullness over the anterior aspect of the joint, since the distribution of the synovial membranes is more extensive in this area (Figs. 14-2 and 14-11). Mild swelling of this joint may not be apparent on inspection but can often be detected by careful palpation. Posterior swelling of the ankle joint in the depression between the malleoli and the Achilles tendon may be difficult to localize to the ankle joint because of other structures in this area that may be involved separately or pushed out by an underlying synovitis of the ankle joint. Thus, it is necessary to differentiate the superficial, linear swelling localized to the distribution of tendon sheaths from the more diffuse fullness and swelling due to involvement of the ankle joint. Synovitis of the intertarsal joints may occasionally cause an erythematous puffiness or fullness over the dorsum of the foot.

Inflammation of ligaments that hold the fore part of the foot together may result in weakening and laxity of the supporting ligamentous structures. When this occurs, the metatarsals and toes spread, and the width of the fore part of the foot is increased. Metatarsal spread thus occurs in some patients with rheumatoid arthritis and often is associated with the more conspicuous findings of hallux valgus and synovitis of the metatarsophalangeal joints. A resulting increase in thickness of the fore part of the foot may keep all or some of the toes from touching the floor when the patient is sitting with the feet in a resting position (Fig. 14–13).

Complete or partial rupture of the Achilles tendon is sudden and dramatic and usually occurs during a burst of unaccustomed physical activity. Pain, swelling, ecchymosis, and tenderness are present at the site of the tear, but the swelling may become more diffuse and include the region of the ankle joint. Tenderness over the Achilles tendon, a visible depression in the tendon at the site of the separation, and pain with, or inability to achieve, flexion of the foot against resistance help in the recognition of this condition.

Abnormal Positions of the Foot

Inspection of the foot may reveal lowering of the longitudinal arch (pes valgoplanus or flatfoot) or abnormal elevation of the longitudinal

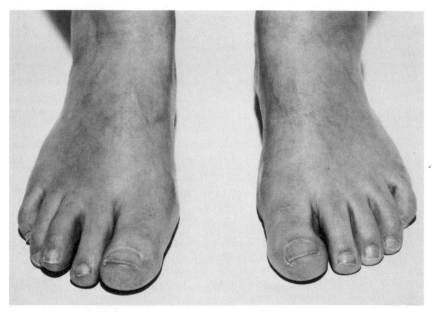

Figure 14–13. Synovitis of the second and third metatarsophalangeal joints of the right foot of a patient with rheumatoid arthritis. Note that the right third toe is raised from the floor level of the other toes and the right second and third toes are spread apart more than any of the other toes. There also is swelling on the dorsum of the right forefoot, although this is less conspicuous than the other abnormalities.

arch (pes cavus). Talipes equinus is the position of the foot in plantar flexion and often results from contracture of the Achilles tendon with elevation of the heel and depression of the fore part of the foot (Fig. 14–12). This tends to occur in bedridden patients. The presence of varus or valgus of the heel is determined by noting deviation of the foot to either side of an imaginary vertical line along the longitudinal axis of the lower extremity. Normally, if this vertical line is dropped from the middle of the patella, it should fall between the first and second toes. Inversion of the foot (supination) exists when the sole of the foot is turned inward, and eversion of the foot (pronation) exists when the sole of the foot is turned outward. Adduction of the foot is present when the fore part of the foot is displaced inward in relation to the midline of the leg. Abduction of the foot occurs when the fore part of the foot is displaced outward in relation to the midline of the limb. The positions of adduction and inversion (varus) or abduction and eversion (valgus) are often combined in deformities of the foot. These abnormalities of the ankles and feet may be associated with abnormalities of the knee such as genu varum (bowlegs) or genu valgum (knock knees).

Abnormal Gaits Associated with Deformities of the Foot

Toe-Out Gait.   A toe-out gait, associated with an outward displacement of the fore part of the foot in relation to the midline of the leg, may develop in patients with abnormalities of the foot and ankle. Patients with painful ankles or feet may splint movement of the foot and ankle by lateral deviation of the foot. This enables the patient to walk by rolling the foot from the lateral to the medial side; this replaces the normal heel-and-toe rolling gait and avoids painful motion in the ankle and joints of the foot. This lateral deviation of the foot often results in an eversion deformity, with the talus and navicular bones being displaced medially and downward and the longitudinal arch dropping so that the patient tends to walk on the inner aspect of his foot. Thus the foot assumes a flat position, and if there is arthritic involvement of the intertarsal joints, the foot may become stiff and rigid. With the foot rotated externally, walking tends to result in increased pressure over the first metatarsophalangeal joint, with weight rolling off the side of the big toe in such a manner as to push it further into a more severe hallux valgus deformity. The eversion and lateral deviation of the foot tend to exert additional strain on the medial ligaments of the knee and thus may force the knee into a genu valgum (knock-knee) position. The toe-out gait is awkward and fatiguing. The abnormalities just described are commonly found in feet affected by rheumatoid arthritis but also may occur in persons without evidence of this disease.

Toe-In Gait.   The toe-in or pigeon-toed gait is the result of an inward displacement of the fore part of the foot in relation to the midline of the lower extremity and is often congenital in origin. This deformity increases weight-bearing on the outer side of the foot, lessening pressure on the first metatarsophalangeal joint. The inward deviation of the fore part of the foot in this condition is often associated with inversion of the foot (supination).

Tarsal Coalition. Tarsal coalition describes a bony, cartilaginous, or fibrous bridging between tarsal bones. It may be associated with deformity of the foot because of related defective growth and development of the foot and with a painful, rigid, pronated gait because of lack of motion between the involved bones and spasm of the adjacent muscles. Inability to stand or walk with feet inverted (soles facing each other) is a physical sign of this condition.

Abnormal Conditions of the Toes

Hallux Valgus. The most common deformity of the great toe is hallus valgus (Fig. 14–14). Hallux valgus is a lateral or outward deviation of the great toe resulting in an abnormal angulation and rotation at the first metatarsophalangeal joint. The first metatarsal bone deviates medially, increases the width of the fore part of the foot and produces a prominence of the first metatarsal head. A callus and bursal reaction are commonly found over this prominence on the medial aspect of the great toe at the metatarsophalangeal joint. If the hallux valgus deformity of the great toe is marked, the big toe may overlap or underlie the second toe.

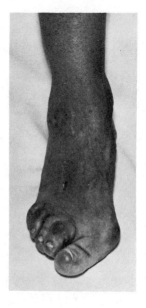

Figure 14–14. Hallux valgus deformity of great toe with spread of the fore part of the foot and a bursal reaction over the medial aspect of the first metatarsophalangeal joint. Hammer-toe deformities with corns are present in the second, third, fourth, and fifth toes.

Limitation of motion at the first metatarsophalangeal joint is called "hallux rigidus."

Hammer Toes, Cockup Toes, and Other Deformities of Toes. The typical hammer-toe deformity consists of hyperextension at the metatarsophalangeal joint, flexion at the proximal interphalangeal joint, and extension of the distal interphalangeal joint and produces a clawlike appearance (Figs. 14–11 and 14–14). However, in some instances the distal interphalangeal joint remains straight, and the tip of the toe touches the floor; this condition is sometimes referred to as "mallet toe." A callus or corn often develops over the prominence of the proximal interphalangeal joint. The second toe is the digit most often involved in a hammer-toe deformity and frequently is associated with a hallux valgus deformity of the big toe.

A cockup deformity of the toe consists of dorsal displacement of the proximal phalanx on the metatarsal head. The metatarsal head becomes depressed toward the sole of the foot, where it can be readily palpated. This deformity causes the tip of the toe to be elevated above the surface on which the foot is resting (Fig. 14–15). A cockup toe represents subluxation of the metatarsophalangeal joint and is associated with arthritic involvement of the metatarsophalangeal joint, whereas the more common hammer toe may occur with or without arthritic involvement of the foot.

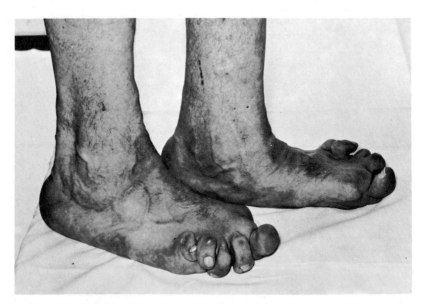

Figure 14–15. Cockup deformities of the toes due to subluxation of the metatarsophalangeal joints in the fourth and fifth toes of each foot. The longitudinal arch is flat in both feet and there is eversion (pronation) of the left foot caused by abnormality of the subtalar joint. This patient has rheumatoid arthritis with involvement and resulting deformities of the other metatarsophalangeal joints.

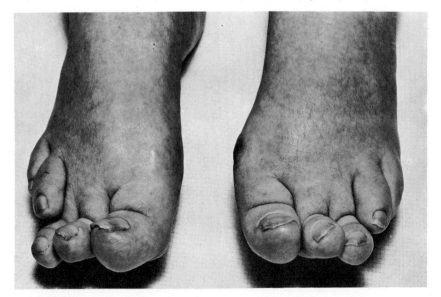

Figure 14–16. Severe hyperextension deformities associated with subluxation of the interphalangeal joints in the first, second, and third toes of each foot due to rheumatoid arthritis, resulting in flail toes.

There also may be lateral displacement of the proximal phalanx on the metatarsal head in any of the toes like that in the big toe with a hallux valgus deformity. This lateral deviation of the toes occurs in a manner similar to ulnar deviation of the fingers in the hand and sometimes results in overlapping of the toes on each other.

Hammer-toe and cockup-toe deformities, or various combinations of the two, often are the result of articular damage and inflammatory changes in the articular capsule and surrounding ligaments of the metatarsophalangeal joints of the second, third, fourth, and fifth toes. Severe articular damage of the interphalangeal joints of the toes may produce hyperextension deformities of the phalanges of the toes (Fig. 14–16).

PALPATION

The Ankle Joint

With the patient seated or supine, the patient's right foot is supported by the examiner's right hand while the fingers of the examiner's left hand palpate the soft tissues overlying the anterior aspect of the joint (Figs. 14–17 and 14–18). The right hand grasps the heel snugly and compresses the area behind and beneath the medial malleolus with the palm and thenar muscles, while the fingers of the same hand apply firm pressure behind and beneath the lateral malleolus in order to distend the

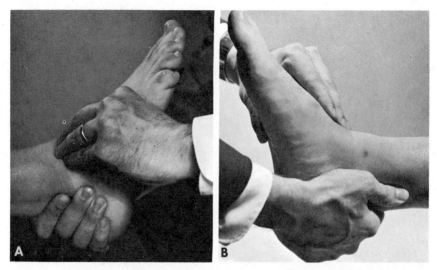

Figure 14–17. Palpation of the ankle. *A.* Lateral aspect of right foot. *B.* Medial aspect of right foot. The patient's foot is supported by the examiner's right hand. With this hand the examiner firmly compresses the posterior aspect of the articular capsule and synovial membrane in order to distend the articular capsule and synovial membrane anteriorly where they can be palpated by the fingers of the examiner's left hand if synovitis is present. See text for details.

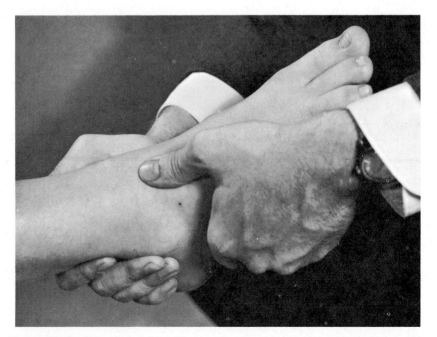

Figure 14–18. Palpation of the ankle when the examiner uses his thumb instead of his fingers. The patient's foot is supported with one hand as described for Figure 14–17, while the thumb of the examiner's other hand palpates over the anterior aspect of the joint to detect tenderness and soft-tissue swelling in this area.

articular capsule and synovial membrane anteriorly, where they can be palpated more easily with the examiner's other hand if synovitis is present in the ankle. Then the fingers or thumb of the examiner's left hand may palpate lightly over the depressed area of the joint space on the anterior aspect of the joint to detect abnormal fullness or soft-tissue swelling in this area. If synovial swelling or effusion of the ankle joint is present, it is most likely to be palpable anteriorly, since the reflection of the synovial membrane is more extensive over the anterior aspect of the joint than elsewhere (Fig. 14–2). It may be difficult to outline the margins of a distended synovial membrane with certainty in this area owing to the presence of overlying structures. Care should be taken to avoid stretching the skin and soft tissues on the anterior aspect of the ankle with the hand that is positioned posteriorly, since the resulting tightness of the skin may make deep palpation and the detection of synovitis more difficult or impossible. The anterior aspect of the ankle may be examined also by using both thumbs, as shown in Figure 14–19. At times, particularly in cases of acute or subacute swelling of the ankle joint, the effusion may be palpated best medially and laterally, between the extensor retinaculum and either malleolus. Occasionally, when the synovium is thin, the fluid can be moved from one side of the ankle to the other by ballottement.

To examine the left foot, the examiner holds the foot with his left hand, palpates with the right hand, and otherwise proceeds as just described.

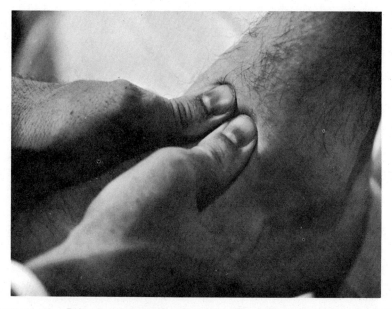

Figure 14–19. Palpation of the ankle (alternate method). The left foot is supported by the fingers of both hands. Both thumbs are used to palpate firmly (note blanched nails) over the anterior aspect of the ankle joint.

Warmth and tenderness may be increased over the ankle joint, but if they are due to synovitis in this area, they should be localized to or maximal in the involved region.

The Heel

A painful heel may be caused by an osseous spur or spurs, inflammation in the Achilles tendon, a calcaneal bursa, or a calcaneal fat pad. Painful heels also may be caused by fractures, osteomyelitis, periostitis, bone tumors, strain on the attachment of the plantar fascia, or other trauma to ligaments and soft tissues about the heels. Careful localization of swelling and tenderness by palpation may help reveal abnormalities in any of these structures.

The Achilles tendon is subject to localized inflammatory reactions and trauma. Palpable swelling and tenderness on the back of the heel may result from inflammation of superficial structures, such as a subcutaneous bursa, or from inflammation of deeper structures, such as the bursa that lies between the calcaneus and the Achilles tendon just proximal to the point of its attachment (Fig. 14–5). It may be difficult to distinguish the more superficial swelling about the tendon from the deeper bursal reaction. However, differentiation of these sites of involvement by palpation is important, when possible, since the deeper bursal reaction often signifies inflammation due to a systemic disease such as rheumatoid arthritis or, rarely, ankylosing spondylitis, whereas the more superficial swelling of an injured tendon or a subcutaneous bursa is often caused by trauma or excessive friction from a tight shoe. An inflamed bursa in the region of the Achilles tendon is often associated with thickness of the skin overlying the bursa, forming a callus. Xanthomatous, tophaceous, fibrous, or rheumatoid nodules may be palpable in the affected part of the tendon. In rupture of the Achilles tendon a defect in the tendon may be palpable. If the tear in the tendon is complete, squeezing the calf while the patient is lying prone with both feet over the edge of the examining table will fail to cause plantar flexion of the foot. Rupture of the Achilles tendon may be confused with thrombophlebitis or with rupture of the plantaris tendon or of fibers of the gastrocnemius muscle. Careful definition of the clinical features and of the structures involved, however, will help in the differentiation.

Pain and tenderness associated with periostitis, seen occasionally in such diseases as Reiter's syndrome and ankylosing spondylitis, may be localized or diffuse over much of the calcaneus.

A self-limited syndrome of pain in the heel occurs with weight-bearing in some adolescents. The symptoms are frequently unilateral. The cause is unknown, but the pain has been attributed to calcaneal epiphysitis and tenosynovitis of the Achilles tendon at the level of its insertion into the os calcis. There is no swelling, but tenderness localized to the posterior superior portion of the os calcis can be discovered by direct and lateral pressure of the examiner's fingers.

Pain on the sole of the foot near the heel may be due to inflammation or trauma at the site of bursae or the attachment of the plantar fascia to the calcaneus (Fig. 14–5). Localized tenderness to palpation over the plantar aspects of the bony prominence of the calcaneus may result from a bursal reaction located between the calcaneus and the skin.

Pain and tenderness under the anterior portion of the heel (often extending into the sole) in the absence of any generalized disorder is frequently called *plantar fasciitis*. It is commonly attributed to occupations that entail excessive standing or walking, especially when the patient is unaccustomed to such an activity, but is not limited to such circumstances, and an exact etiology may not be recognized. In such patients, roentgenograms may or may not reveal a bony spur at the attachment of plantar fascia to the calcaneus. The two most common sites for spurs in the heel are: (1) the plantar surface of the calcaneus near the site of attachment of the plantar fascia and (2) the insertion of the Achilles tendon in the posterior aspect of the calcaneus (Fig. 14–5). The pain associated with calcaneal spurs is due primarily to the inflammatory reaction in adjacent soft tissues rather than to the bony spur itself. Calcaneal spurs are frequently asymptomatic and may be seen in a lateral roentgenogram of the foot.

Intertarsal Joints

The intertarsal joints are palpated distal to the ankle between the examiner's thumbs on the dorsum of the foot and his fingers on the plantar surface of the foot. Swelling, tenderness, and warmth are the main physical findings that may be detected by palpation. Usually these signs are present on the dorsal rather than the plantar aspect of the foot. Although tenderness may be localized, swelling is rarely localized to any particular intertarsal joint (except occasionally the talocalcaneonavicular joint), and it usually is detected as generalized thickening or fullness over the dorsum of the foot. Swelling in this region must be differentiated from localized tenosynovitis of the extensors of the foot.

Metatarsophalangeal Joints

The metatarsophalangeal joints are palpated between the examiner's thumb and forefinger, as shown in Figure 14–20. The thumb is placed on the dorsum of the foot, and the fingers of the same hand are positioned on the plantar aspect about 0.5 cm proximal to the position of the thumb in order to locate the metatarsal heads.

The examiner palpates the metatarsal heads on both the dorsal

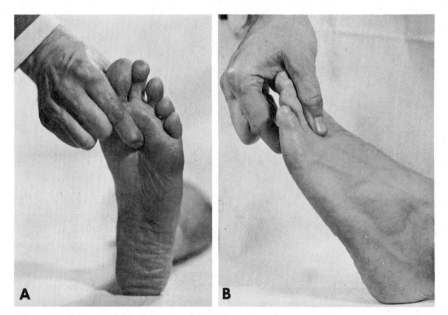

Figure 14–20. Palpation of metatarsophalangeal joints of left foot. *A.* Plantar view. *B.* Lateral view. The forefinger is palpating deeply between the second and third metatarsal heads. Note how far proximally the metatarsal heads actually are located. See text for details.

and plantar aspects of the foot but especially through the soft tissues over the plantar surface. The soft tissues on the plantar aspect consist of thick skin, superficial fascia, and adipose tissue. The fascia and adipose tissue serve as a padding between the bones and skin in addition to the underlying articular capsule and the synovial membrane of the metatarsophalangeal joints. The soft-tissue thickness varies with the amount of synovitis and with the thickness or atrophy of the fat pads and other subcutaneous tissues. Palpation over the metatarsal heads not only gives information about the soft-tissue reactions in this area but also may reveal deformities or subluxation in the metatarsophalangeal joints. Subluxation of a metatarsophalangeal joint produces a dorsal displacement of the proximal phalanx on the metatarsal head, and the metatarsal head becomes more than usually prominent on the plantar aspect of the foot, where it can be palpated easily. Subluxation of a metatarsophalangeal joint commonly produces a cockup deformity of the toe, as described in the paragraphs on "Inspection."

In the presence of chronic synovitis (for example, rheumatoid arthritis) involving the metatarsophalangeal joints and supporting ligaments, there is a loss of the normal fat pad under the metatarsal bones, and spreading of the metatarsals is likely. When the soft-tissue reaction and swelling subside, the metatarsal heads lie directly under the skin, where they are readily palpable and are also subject to additional trauma.

Palpation for synovitis of the metatarsophalangeal joints is performed by starting proximally between the shafts of any two adjacent metatarsal bones. As the thumb and fingers of the examiner are gradually moved distally toward the metatarsophalangeal joint, the area between the metatarsal bones is palpated. Normally, the palpating finger can extend a short distance into the groove between adjacent metatarsal bones and the groove between adjacent metatarsal heads. However, the second and third metatarsal bones are tightly bound together in the normal individual, so that it is normally difficult to palpate between them satisfactorily. The region over the metatarsal head and the groove between adjacent metatarsal heads are firmly palpated for evidence of synovial thickening or distention by rolling the examining forefinger over and between the plantar surfaces of the metatarsal heads (Fig. 14–20). Normally, the synovial membrane cannot be palpated in the groove between adjacent metatarsal heads but, in the presence of boggy synovial thickening or distention, this groove may be partially obliterated by the abnormal distribution or reaction of the synovial membrane. Lesser degrees of synovial thickening of one or more metatarsophalangeal joints may be more easily detected on the dorsal surface by palpating the joint margins with one hand, as shown in Figure 14–20, and by making simultaneous comparisons by examining the opposite foot with the other hand. Palpable swelling and tenderness between any two adjacent metatarsophalangeal joints may represent a local inflammatory process accompanying a neuroma or may represent synovial swelling in the metatarsophalangeal joint. The soft-tissue swelling of synovitis is palpable on both sides of the involved joint.

Tenderness to palpation over the metatarsophalangeal joint is particularly helpful in detecting abnormal involvement of this joint and is often present when there is synovitis in the joint, but local heat or redness is usually absent. Tenderness of the metatarsophalangeal joints can be evaluated by firmly palpating each joint between the thumb and the forefinger (Fig. 14–20) and also (but with less localization) by grasping the fore part of the patient's foot with one hand and squeezing the metatarsal heads together between the thumb on one side of the foot and the fingers on the other side.

Interphalangeal Joints

The proximal and distal interphalangeal joints of the toes are palpated in a manner similar to palpation of the corresponding joints in the fingers. The examiner's thumb and forefinger are used to palpate the medial and lateral aspect of the joint (Fig. 14–21). Synovitis in the interphalangeal joints is usually detected best on the medial and lateral aspects of the joint while varying degrees of pressure are applied by the palpating fingers to determine the presence of swelling, tenderness, or warmth.

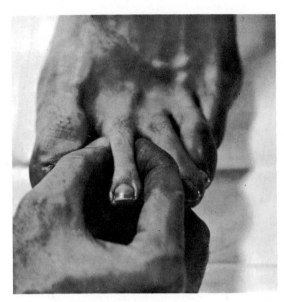

Figure 14–21. Palpation of the proximal interphalangeal joint of the left second toe. The examiner's thumb and forefinger are used to palpate the medial and lateral aspects of the joint to detect swelling and tenderness.

Other Abnormalities of the Foot and Ankle

Tenosynovitis Near the Ankle. The tendons crossing the region of the ankle are enclosed for part of their course in synovial sheaths, as described on page 240. When these synovial tendon sheaths become inflamed (tenosynovitis), it is important to differentiate the superficial linear swelling and tenderness of tenosynovitis from the more generalized swelling and fullness of synovitis in the underlying ankle joint. The swelling and tenderness of tenosynovitis can be localized by palpation over the distribution of the tendon sheaths, whereas the swelling and tenderness of synovitis in the ankle joint when palpated anteriorly is found in the distribution of the synovial membrane over the anterior aspect of the joint. At times the swelling of the tendon sheath is obscured by a more diffuse overlying edema, but when the edema is reduced by rest in bed and elevation of the extremity, careful palpation may show that the deeper swelling and tenderness follow the line of the tendon. Tenosynovitis frequently causes pain on movement of the involved tendon. Thus, inversion or eversion of the foot against resistance may cause pain when there is a tenosynovial reaction on the respective medial or lateral aspect of the foot or ankle, and extension of the foot against resistance may be painful when there is a tenosynovial reaction of the extensor tendons on the anterior portion of the ankle. However, failure to produce pain with these maneuvers does not exclude a tenosynovial reaction.

The most commonly involved tendons are the posterior tibial, peroneal, extensor digitorum longus, and anterior tibial tendons. Figure 14-22*A* shows a conspicuous example of tenosynovitis of the Achilles tendon sheath in a patient with severe rheumatoid arthritis; Figure 14-22*B* shows posterior tibial tenosynovitis.

Metatarsalgia. Metatarsalgia, or pain and tenderness of the plantar surface of the heads of the metatarsal bones or of the metatarsophalangeal joints, is a common complaint that occurs alone or in association with many local and systemic conditions. In youth, trauma and osteochondritis of the second metatarsal head are common causes. In the adult, any disturbance that can affect the feet (for example, circulatory, neurogenic, infectious, rheumatic, or traumatic) can first manifest itself in the metatarsal region of one or both feet. When there is no specifically relatable condition, the middle metatarsal heads often can be shown to bear a disproportionate amount of weight. In such "static" instances, callus develops under one or more of the heads of the second, third, or fourth metatarsals.

Interdigital Neuroma (Morton's Toe). Interdigital neuroma must be differentiated from metatarsalgia, just described. An interdigital neuroma is a fusiform enlargement of an interdigital nerve that is most commonly located between or distal to the heads of the third and fourth metatarsal bones. It is usually unilateral and more common in women. Pain, which is sharp or burning in quality, occurs first with activity and later also at rest. A typical feature is the history of relief of pain obtained by the patient when the shoe is removed and the foot massaged. Sharply localized tenderness is characteristic and is present in the soft, fleshy tissue either between or distal to the heads of the third and fourth metatarsals (less often of the second and third). The location of the tenderness can differentiate it from tenderness of the metatarsophalangeal joint. Altered sensation may be found on the lateral aspect of the third toe and medial aspect of the fourth toe. Occasionally, a large interdigital neuroma may be palpated and found to be movable between the heads of the metatarsals.

March Foot. The march foot is caused by severe or prolonged use of the foot, such as during strenuous marching, and usually results in a transverse fracture of a metatarsal shaft. The second metatarsal is affected most frequently and the third metatarsal next most frequently, but any of the metatarsals can be involved. Localized pain develops over the dorsum of the fore part of the foot, causing the patient to limp. The most common and significant findings on physical examination are palpable tenderness and swelling over the fracture The diagnosis is confirmed by roentgenographic examination or bone scan of the foot. Stress fractures also may occur in the calcaneus or the lower part of the tibia or fibula.

Reflex Sympathetic Dystrophy (Sudek's Atrophy). Reflex sympathetic dystrophy is an incompletely understood syndrome that in-

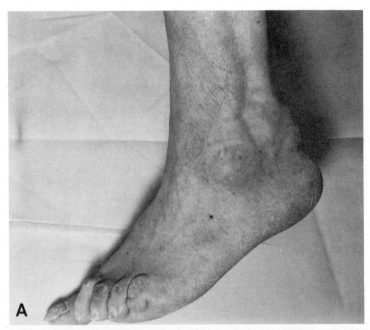

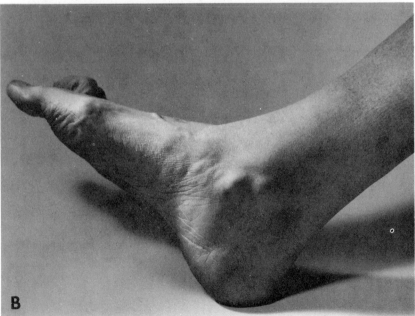

Figure 14–22. *See legend on opposite page.*

volves the entire foot and ankle and easily can be mistaken for, or associated with, an atypical polyarthritis. It can be a sequel to, or complication of, trauma, but it frequently has no obvious or detectable organic cause. The foot typically is cyanotic or mottled, edematous, tender, cool, moist, and shiny. Hyperalgesia, although present, often does not conform to any definitive anatomic structural distribution. Pain may be mild at rest, and the discomfort, other than in cases of hyperalgesia or paresthesia, may be less than would be expected with a comparable degree of arthritis. Weight-bearing is very painful and is usually resisted or avoided.

When it involves the foot, the syndrome of transient osteoporosis of the lower extremities is similar to reflex dystrophy. Tenderness of the tarsal and metatarsal bones is present, and weight-bearing is painful. In transient osteoporosis, however, the color of the skin is usually normal, swelling tends to be minimal, recurrences are common, and the knee or hip may be involved.

Tarsal Tunnel Syndrome (Posterior Tibial Nerve Entrapment). As the posterior tibial nerve reaches the ankle joint, it passes behind and under the medial malleolus and beneath the flexor retinaculum (Fig. 14–3). The flexor retinaculum forms a roof over the bony hollow behind the medial malleolus and thereby converts the region into a fibro-osseous canal, the tarsal tunnel, which is somewhat analogous anatomically to the carpal tunnel at the wrist. In its passage through the tarsal tunnel, the posterior tibial nerve is accompanied by the posterior tibial and flexor digitorum longus tendons and the posterior tibial artery and veins anteriorly and by the flexor hallucis longus tendon posteriorly. As the posterior tibial nerve enters the tunnel, one or two calcaneal branches of the nerve emerge above or through the flexor retinaculum to innervate the skin on the medial aspect of the heel. In the tunnel or just beyond it, the posterior tibial nerve divides into the medial and lateral plantar branches. These innervate the intrinsic muscles of the foot and supply sensory branches to the sole of the foot and the toes. The medial branch contains sensory fibers for the medial aspect of the sole, the medial three toes, and the medial aspect of the fourth toe; the lateral plan-

---

Figure 14–22. *A.* Tenosynovitis of the Achilles tendon sheath in a patient with severe rheumatoid arthritis. The ankle joint is not affected, as may be noted by the absence of swelling anteriorly over the joint, but the metatarsophalangeal joints have subluxed and resulted in hammer-toe deformities of the second, third, fourth, and fifth toes. The Achilles tenosynovitis may be contrasted with its absence in the patient's foot shown in *B. B.* Chronic tenosynovitis of the posterior tibial tendon sheath in a patient with rheumatoid arthritis. The swelling is most conspicuous both below and distal to the medial malleolus, where the tendon and its sheath are relatively more superficial. The involvement may be contrasted with its absence in the patient's foot pictured in *A.* Also note the absence of evidence of synovitis of the ankle joint.

tar nerve supplies the lateral half of the sole, the lateral aspect of the fourth toe, and all of the fifth toe.

Excess accumulation of fat, tenosynovitis, fibrosis, fixation of the nerve due to bone or joint deformity, trauma such as fracture, strain during pronation, or an external chronic trauma that might occur secondary to ill-fitting shoes (often associated with posterior tibial tendinitis) can produce symptoms of the tarsal tunnel syndrome. Hypertrophy of the abductor hallucis muscle, chronic compression from fascial bands, and venous varicosities also have been found in reported cases. However, this condition is quite uncommon except when it is secondary to trauma affecting the area.

Characteristic symptoms of the tarsal tunnel syndrome are burning pain, tingling, or numbness in the toes, forefoot, or heel in the distribution of the particular branch or branches entrapped. When severe, the discomfort also may extend into the calf. Symptoms are frequently most pronounced in the toes and distal part of the sole. The discomfort may be constant or intermittent and is typically accentuated by prolonged standing and walking. Occasionally a crampy pain or sensation of tightness is noted on the sole of the foot. If the calcaneal branches are involved, the symptoms will be in the medial plantar surface of the heel and may mimic those of a calcaneal spur.

The physical signs include tenderness along the nerve in the tarsal tunnel or distal to it. Tinel's sign may be elicited in some instances over the posterior tibial nerve at the site of compression by using the same technique as that used to demonstrate medial nerve compression at the wrist (see p. 110). Decreased sensation to pinprick or to two-point discrimination is found earlier and more commonly than motor weakness or atrophy of the flexors of the toes or the abductor hallucis. Electromyographic measurement may show an increase in the conduction time of the entrapped nerve.

MOVEMENT AND RANGE OF MOTION

Movement at the ankle (talocrural) joint is limited almost entirely to plantar flexion and dorsiflexion. From the normal position of rest in which there is an angle of 90 degrees between the leg and foot (labeled 0 degrees in Figure 14-23), the ankle joint normally allows about 20 degrees of dorsiflexion and about 45 degrees of plantar flexion.

Inversion and eversion of the foot occur mainly at the subtalar (subastragalar) and other intertarsal articulations. Inversion of the foot (supination) exists when the sole of the foot is turned inward, and eversion of the foot (pronation) exists when the sole of the foot is turned outward. From the normal position of rest, the subtalar joint normally

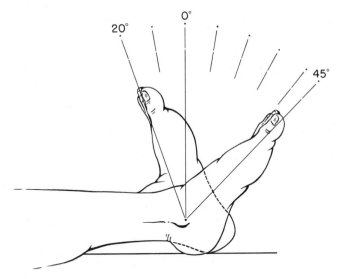

Figure 14-23. Normal range of plantar flexion (0 to 45 degrees) and dorsiflexion (0 to 20 degrees) in ankle joint.

permits about 20 degrees of eversion and about 30 degrees of inversion (Fig. 14–24). To examine the specific movements of the subtalar joint, the examiner first dorsiflexes the ankle joint to the neutral position (0 degrees, Fig. 14–23) to prevent lateral movement of the talus at the ankle joint. Then the calcaneus is gripped and the foot is moved into inversion and eversion. The patient should be relaxed or even actively assist the movement. To examine the movements of the midtarsal joints, the examiner holds the calcaneus in one hand and the forefoot in the other and rotates the midfoot in both directions in relation to the calcaneus, then compares the range of motion in each foot.

Muscle weakness, synovitis, tarsal coalition, and stretching of inflamed ligaments in the midportion of the foot and in the region of the intertarsal joints may be associated with characteristic deformities and limitation of motion in the foot. A condition known as pes planovalgus is said to be the most common midtarsal deformity in patients with rheumatoid arthritis.

The metatarsophalangeal joint of the great toe extends (dorsiflexion) about 80 degrees and flexes (plantar flexion) about 35 degrees (Fig. 14–25). The metatarsophalangeal joints of the second to fifth toes move only about 40 degrees in either flexion or extension. The proximal interphalangeal joints normally do not extend beyond the position indicated by 0 degrees, but do flex about 50 degrees (Fig. 14–26). In the distal interphalangeal joints, extension varies in the different toes but may be as much as 30 degrees, and flexion is about 40 to 50 degrees.

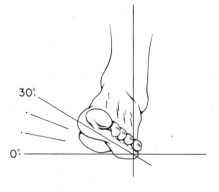

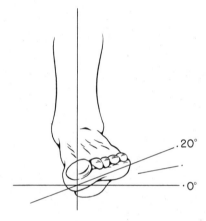

Figure 14–24. Normal range of inversion (supination, 0 to 30 degrees) and eversion (pronation, 0 to 20 degrees) in subtalar joint.

Figure 14–25. Normal range of extension (dorsiflexion) in the first metatarsophalangeal joint (0 to 80 degrees) and normal range of flexion (plantar flexion) in second to fifth metatarsophalangeal joints (0 to 35 degrees).

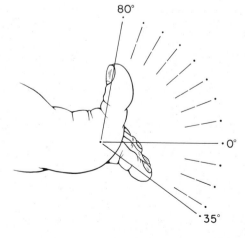

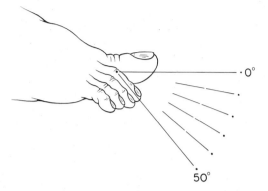

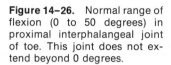

Figure 14-26. Normal range of flexion (0 to 50 degrees) in proximal interphalangeal joint of toe. This joint does not extend beyond 0 degrees.

0°

50°

MUSCLE TESTING

Joints of the Ankle and Foot

Plantar Flexion of the Ankle. The prime movers in plantar flexion of the ankle are the gastrocnemius (tibial nerve, S1,2) and the soleus (tibial nerve, S1,2) muscles. The tibialis posterior, peroneus longus, peroneus brevis, flexor hallucis longus, flexor digitorum longus, and plantaris muscles are accessory to this motion. The tibialis posterior, peroneus longus, and peroneus brevis muscles must be strong enough to stabilize the forefoot during flexion of the ankle. Plantar flexion of the ankle is tested with the patient standing on the leg to be tested, with the knee straight. The patient is instructed to raise the heel from the floor through its range of motion, lifting the weight of the body. If muscle strength is normal, the patient is able to raise the heel repeatedly. Alternatively, if the patient can walk on his toes the muscle strength of the plantar flexors of the ankle can be considered normal. Plantar flexion can also be tested with the patient lying supine with the lower extremity extended and a pad under the knee to prevent hyperextension. The examiner holds the leg proximal to the ankle against the table with one hand to stabilize the leg. The patient then flexes the foot against graded resistance provided by the examiner's other hand, which grasps and holds the calcaneus and exerts pressure against the pull of the plantar flexors. The examiner may need to exert counterpressure with the forearm against the sole of the foot if the accessory muscles that stabilize the forefoot are functioning, as shown in Figure 14-27.

Dorsiflexion and Inversion of the Foot. The prime mover in dorsiflexion and inversion of the foot is the tibialis anterior muscle (deep peroneal nerve, L4,5, S1). Dorsiflexion and inversion of the foot are tested while the patient sits with legs over the edge of the table. The examiner holds the leg above the ankle with one hand to immobilize it. The patient then dorsiflexes and inverts the foot while keeping the toes relaxed or flexed. The examiner uses his other hand to apply graded resis-

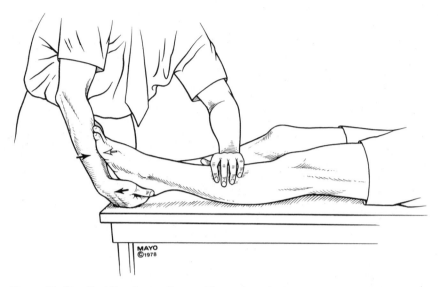

Figure 14–27. Test for plantar flexors. The patient, in the supine position, flexes the ankle. The examiner holds the leg with one hand to stabilize it and provides resistance against flexion with the other hand by holding the calcaneus and exerting counter-pressure with the forearm against the patient's foot. A pad may be placed under the knee to prevent hyperextension.

tance on the medial and dorsal aspects of the foot, as shown in Figure 14–28. If the big toe is not relaxed or flexed, substitution by the extensor hallucis longus muscle may interfere with the proper evaluation of the test. Alternatively, if the patient can walk on his heels, the muscular strength of the foot in dorsiflexion can be considered normal.

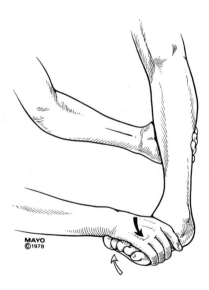

Figure 14–28. Test for dorsiflexion and inversion of the foot. The patient, in a sitting position, dorsiflexes and inverts the foot. The examiner stabilizes the leg with one hand and provides resistance to flexion and inversion with the other hand on the forefoot.

Inversion of the Foot.   The prime mover in inversion of the foot is the tibialis posterior muscle (tibial nerve, L5, S1). The flexor digitorum longus and flexor hallucis longus muscles and the medial head of the gastrocnemius muscle are accessory to this motion. Inversion of the foot is tested with the patient lying on his side with the foot in plantar flexion. The examiner holds the leg above the ankle with one hand to stabilize the leg. The patient then moves the foot through the range of inversion while the examiner applies graded resistance on the medial border of the forefoot with his other hand.

Eversion of the Foot.   The prime movers in eversion of the foot are the peroneus longus (superficial peroneal nerve, L4,5, S1) and peroneus brevis (superficial peroneal nerve, L4,5, S1) muscles. The extensor digitorum longus and peroneus tertius muscles are accessory to this motion. Eversion of the foot is tested while the patient is lying on his side, as just described for testing inversion. The examiner holds the leg above the ankle with one hand to stabilize it. The patient then everts the foot against graded resistance applied by the examiner's other hand over the lateral aspect of the foot. The peroneus brevis is tested while graded resistance is applied to the lateral border of the foot near the insertion of this muscle at the base of the fifth metatarsal. The peroneus longus is tested while graded resistance is applied to the plantar surface of the first metatarsal head near its insertion at the base of the first metatarsal.

Joints of the First Toe

Flexion of the Metatarsophalangeal Joint.   The prime mover in flexion of this joint is the flexor hallucis brevis muscle (medial plantar nerve, L4,5, S1). The flexor hallucis longus muscle is accessory to this motion. Flexion of the first metatarsophalangeal joint is tested while the patient is supine and legs are extended. The examiner holds the patient's foot in the midtarsal region with one hand to stabilize the metatarsal bones. The patient then flexes the first toe while attempting to avoid flexion of the interphalangeal joint, and the examiner provides graded resistance to flexion with his other hand beneath the first proximal phalanx.

Flexion of the Interphalangeal Joint.   The prime mover of flexion of this joint is the flexor hallucis longus muscle (tibial nerve, L5, S1,2). Flexion of the interphalangeal joint of the first toe is tested while the proximal phalanx of the toe is stabilized between the thumb and index finger of one of the examiner's hands. The patient flexes the interphalangeal joint against graded resistance provided by one or more fingers of the examiner's other hand beneath the distal phalanx of the first toe.

Extension of the Metatarsophalangeal and Interphalangeal Joints.   The prime mover in extension of the metatarsophalangeal joint of the first toe is the medial division of the extensor digitorum brevis muscle (deep peroneal nerve, L5, S1). Extension of this joint is performed while the examiner stabilizes the metatarsal bone of the toe between the thumb and fingers of one hand. The patient then extends the metatarsophalangeal joint against graded manual resistance provided over the dorsal surface of the proximal phalanx by the examiner. The prime mover in extension of the interphalangeal joint of the first toe is the extensor hallucis longus muscle (deep peroneal nerve, L4,5, S1). Extension of the interphalangeal joint of the first toe is tested while the examiner stabilizes the proximal phalanx of the toe between the thumb and index finger of one hand. The patient then extends the distal phalanx against graded resistance provided over the dorsal surface of the phalanx by one or more fingers of the examiner's other hand.

Joints of the Second Through Fifth Toes

Flexion of the Metatarsophalangeal Joints. The prime movers in flexion of the second through fifth metatarsophalangeal joints are the lumbrical muscles (first lumbrical: medial plantar nerve, L4,5; second, third, and fourth lumbricals: lateral plantar nerve, S1,2). The dorsal and plantar interossei, flexor digiti quinti brevis, flexor digitorum longus, and flexor digitorum brevis muscles are accessory to this motion. Flexion of the metatarsophalangeal joints of the second through fifth toes is tested in the same way as described for flexion of the first toe, except that the examiner provides graded resistance to flexion with his other hand beneath the proximal row of phalanges, as shown in Figure 14-29. Individual toes also should be tested separately.

Flexion of the Proximal and Distal Interphalangeal Joints. The prime mover in flexion of the proximal interphalangeal joints of the second through fifth toes is the flexor digitorum brevis muscle (medial plantar nerve, L4,5). Flexion of these joints is tested similarly to flexion of the metatarsophalangeal joints. The examiner stabilizes the proximal row of phalanges of the second through fifth toes by holding them between the thumb and fingers of one hand. The patient then flexes the toes against graded resistance provided by the examiner's other hand beneath the second or middle row of phalanges.

The prime mover in flexion of the distal interphalangeal joints of the second through fifth toes is the flexor digitorum longus muscle (tibial nerve, L5, S1). To test flexion of these joints, the examiner stabilizes the middle row of phalanges of the second through fifth toes by holding them between his thumb and fingers. The patient then flexes the distal phalanges against graded resistance provided by the examiner's other hand beneath the distal phalanges. Because of the shortness of the toes and the usually underdeveloped state of their muscles, it may be difficult to distinguish between flexion at the proximal and distal interphalangeal joints in many persons.

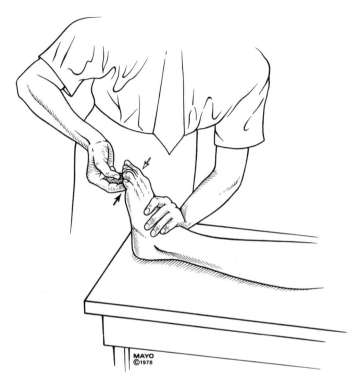

Figure 14-29. Test for flexors of the second through fifth metatarsophalangeal joints. The patient flexes these joints while the examiner holds the foot with one hand to stabilize the metatarsals and provides resistance to flexion with the fingers of the other hand beneath the proximal row of phalanges.

Extension of the Metatarsophalangeal and Interphalangeal Joints. The prime movers in extension of these joints are the extensor digitorum longus (deep peroneal nerve, L4,5, S1) and extensor digitorum brevis (deep peroneal nerve, L5, S1) muscles. Extension of the metatarsophalangeal joints and interphalangeal joints is tested at the same time, while the examiner holds the forefoot with one hand to stabilize the metatarsal bones. The patient then extends the second through fifth toes against resistance provided by the fingers of the examiner's other hand on the dorsal surface of the proximal phalanges. The individual interphalangeal joints cannot usually be tested separately because the extensor digitorum brevis and extensor digitorum longus tendons to the second, third, and fourth digits are fused. Thus, both muscles extend all the joints of these toes. The extensor digitorum longus extends the fifth toe, but the extensor digitorum brevis inserts only on the first four toes. If the extensor digitorum longus is paralyzed, a strong extensor digitorum brevis will extend the metatarsophalangeal joint of the first toe and all the joints of the second, third, and fourth toes. In such instances, palpation of the tendons and muscle bellies will help determine the status of each muscle.

SUGGESTED READING FOR ADDITIONAL INFORMATION

1. Inman VT: The Joints of the Ankle. Baltimore, Williams & Wilkins Company, 1976, 117 pp.
2. Giannestras NJ (editor): Foot Disorders: Medical and Surgical Management. Second edition. Philadelphia, Lea & Febiger, 1973, 699 pp.
3. Inman VT (editor): Du Vries' Surgery of the Foot. Third edition. St. Louis, CV Mosby Company, 1973, 567 pp.

INDEX

References to illustrations are in **boldface** type.
Tables are indicated by *t*.